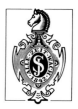

Manuel Viamonte Jr.

Errors in Abdominal Radiology

With 50 Figures in 176 Separate Illustrations

Springer-Verlag
Berlin Heidelberg New York
London Paris Tokyo
Hong Kong Barcelona
Budapest

Prof. Manuel Viamonte Jr., M.D., M.Sc.
Chairman and Director
Department of Radiology
Mount Sinai Medical Center
University of Miami School of Medicine
4300 Alton Road
Miami Beach, FL 33140
USA

ISBN 3-540-54080-6 Springer-Verlag Berlin Heidelberg New York
ISBN 0-387-54080-6 Springer-Verlag New York Berlin Heidelberg

Library of Congress Cataloging-in-Publication Data. Viamonte, Manuel, 1930 –. Errors in abdominal radiology / Manuel Viamonte Jr., p. cm.
ISBN 3-540-54080-6 (alk. paper). – ISBN 0-387-54080-6 (alk. paper)
1. Abdomen-Radiology. 2. Diagnostic errors. I. Title. [DNLM: 1. Abdomen-radiology-atlases 2. Diagnostic Errors-atlases. 3. Gastrointestinal Diseases-diagnosis. WI 900 V613e] RC944.V53 1992 617.5′50757–dc20 DNLM/DLC for Library of Congress 91-4827 CIP

© Springer-Verlag Berlin Heidelberg 1992
Printed in Germany

The use of registered names, trademarks, etc. in this publication does not imply, even in the absence of a specific statement, that such names are exempt from the relevant protective laws and regulations and therefore free for general use.

Product liability: The publishers cannot guarantee the accuracy of any information about dosage and application contained in this book. In every individual case the user must check such information by consulting the relevant literature.

Reproduction of the figures: Gustav Dreher GmbH, Stuttgart, FRG
Typesetting, printed and binding: Konrad Triltsch, Graphischer Betrieb, Würzburg, FRG
21/3130-5 4 3 2 1 0 – Printed on acid-free paper

Acknowledgements

Grateful acknowledgement is given to the following for use of figures in this publication:

Ruby L. Belton, M.D., Northside Radiology, P.C., Rochester, NY, for figures from R.L. Belton and T.F. VanZandt. Congenital Absence of the Left Lobe of the Liver: A Radiologic Diagnosis. Radiology 147:184, April, 1983

Barry Green, M.D., Good Samaritan Regional Medical Center, Phoenix, AZ, for permission to reprint figures from A. Prando, H.M. Goldstein, M.E. Bernardino, and B. Green. Ultrasonic Pseudolesions of the Liver. Radiology 130:403–407, February, 1979

Robert A. Halvorsen, M.D., University of California, San Francisco, CA, for permission to reprint figures from CT Evaluation of Atypical Hepatic Fatty Metamorphosis. J Computer Assisted Tomog, Nov./Dec., 1990

Hedvig Hricak, M.D., University of California, San Francisco, CA, for figure 48

Arthur de Paula Lobo, M.D., Clinica Radiologica de Octavio Lobo, Belem, Brazil, for Fig. 18

Andrew C. Wilbur, M.D., College of Medicine at Chicago, Chicago, IL, for figures from A.C. Wilbur, D.J. Schmit, J.C. Ryva, and S.A. Renigers. Accessory Hepatic Fissure Mimicking an Acoustically Shadowing Lesion. J Ultrasound Med 5:341–342, June, 1986

American Institute of Ultrasound in Medicine for figures from A.C. Wilbur, D.J. Schmit, J.C. Ryva, and S.A. Renigers. Accessory Hepatic Fissure Mimicking an Acoustically Shadowing Lesion. J Ultrasound Med 5:341–342, June, 1986

Mosby Yearbook, Inc., for figures from: A. Margulis and J. Burhenne. Alimentary Tract Roentgenology. C.V. Mosby, St. Louis, 1973

The Radiological Society of North America for permission to reprint figures from R.L. Belton and T.F. VanZandt. Congenital Absence of the Left Lobe of the Liver: A Radiologic Diagnosis. Radiology 147:184, April, 1983

The Radiological Society of North America for permission to reprint figures (Figs. 1 and 2) from A. Prando, H.M. Goldstein, M.E. Bernardino, and B. Green. Ultrasonic Pseudolesions of the Liver. Radiology 130:403–407, February, 1979

Contents

Introduction

There are many diagnostic imaging techniques for the radiological examination of the abdomen. Noninvasive methods include supine and upright views of the abdomen (sometimes fluoroscopy and decubitus films); posteroanterior (PA) views of the chest; contrast studies of the alimentary tract; ultrasonography (US), scintigraphy, computed tomography (CT), and magnetic resonance imaging (MRI). Biopsy under fluoroscopic control and angiography are invasive techniques.

Most of the errors described in this book are related to faulty interpretation; others are due to improper technique. For example, a patient with acute abdominal pain secondary to a perforated hollow viscus may be studied only by supine and upright views of the abdomen that do not include the subdiaphragmatic regions. A complementary PA view of the chest or a left lateral decubitus film would, however, detect free air in the peritoneal cavity that the incomplete two-film study might have missed.

Errors of technique are due to under- or overexposure, long examination times or an uncooperative patient (both of which can induce motion artifacts), improper processing, and failure to perform the proper standard noninvasive or invasive modalities for examining the hollow viscus and the solid organs of the alimentary tract.

In order to visualize the diaphragm and the supra- and infradiaphragmatic spaces, frontal and lateral chest roentgenograms complement the standard views of the abdomen. Fluoroscopy is of great value in assessing diaphragmatic motion as well as being essential when contrast media are utilized. Special filters have been used with variable success to outline the fat − soft tissue interfaces of the flanks.

Supine views of the abdomen can be supplemented with prone frontal views and with both decubitus images. This is particularly important when bowel obstruction or free air in the peritoneal cavity is suspected.

Simple contrast studies include the use of water-soluble, iodine-containing contrast media in cases where perforations are suspected, and complete or limited barium enema examinations when left-sided colonic pathology is suggested by clinical and/or standard radiographic studies.

The radiographic techniques should be varied according to the different organs being examined or the suspected pathology but a consistently high standard should always be achieved.

Interpretation of Radiological Examination

An orderly approach should be taken to interpreting radiological studies to ensure that any significant pathology is detected. The following is suggested, particularly for neophytes:

1. Examine the "four corners of the film" (i.e., costodiaphragmatic angles, supra- and infradiaphragmatic spaces bilaterally). Special attention should be given to the lung bases and hip regions, and in particular to gas shadows that may project below the iliopectineal line. These may simply represent air in the bowel of individuals with a pendulous abdomen, or air in a herniated bowel (e.g., inguinal hernia, which can be discovered by observing air projecting below the iliopectineal line, usually on one side).

2. Evaluate the bony structures (lower thoracic and lumbosacral spine, lower ribs, iliac bones, and proximal femora). Relevant or unsuspected pathology of the spine may be the cause of the patient's symptoms. Occasionally, one may observe destructive lesions of the bony skeleton which will reinforce a preliminary diagnosis of abdominal or extraabdominal malignancy (e.g., a patient with hepatomegaly or some abdominal mass with signs of bony metastasis).

3. Examine the flanks, paying special attention to the fat-muscle interfaces, and look for possible extraluminal air collections.

4. Examine the organs of the alimentary tract, starting with the hollow viscera. a) Focus on the esophagogastric region and then study the stomach, the duodenum, and the small and large bowel sequentially. Rule out intraluminal masses (e.g., cancer of the stomach revealed by an abnormal segment of the stomach where air has been replaced by a mass). Pay attention to the air-containing bowel and evaluate the distribution of air as well as the caliber and contours of the bowel. Occasionally, different forms of colitis or even cancer of the colon can be diagnosed by observing an alteration in the bowel contour. Then, look for the presence of air in the wall of the bowel and extraluminally.

Numerous signs have been described in the literature regarding extraluminal air. These include subdiaphragmatic air, "the cresent sign," triangular and linear gas collections in the right upper quadrant; Rigler's sign, "the wall sign"; the "falciform ligament sign," and the "football sign."

If free air is suspected under the diaphragm, the possibility of fat should always be excluded. The lack of displacement of a curvilinear lucency in the juxtadiaphragmatic region suggests the presence of fat and not air.

There are pitfalls in the interpretation of free air in the peritoneal cavity. These include air within the duodenum simulating free subhepatic air, fat in the region of the ligamentum teres simulating air in that location, and bowel contents with air bubbles simulating an abscess or air in the retroperitoneum.

The small and large bowel can usually be recognized from their anatomy in adults, but in infants it is often difficult to distinguish small from large bowel. Contrast studies may become necessary, particularly in infants, when the small and the large bowel must be delineated and a definite diagnosis of bowel pathology is to be made.

b) Examine *the solid organs,* particularly of the alimentary and genitourinary tract (i.e., liver, spleen, kidneys, and gynecological organs). Study their size, shape, location, and density.

5. Pay attention to abnormal densities, particularly calcifications. Soft tissue densities can be produced by fluid in the bowel or by masses in the region of the kidneys, adrenals, gallbladder, and pelvic organs. A urine-distended bladder can simulate a hypogastric mass. When there is a pelvic mass, it may be necessary to have the patient void, in order to rule out a distended urinary bladder.

Calcific densities can be due to *vascular* structures, such as atherosclerotic lesions in the abdominal aorta, iliac arteries, and femoral arteries, and phleboliths, particularly in the region of the pelvis. When phleboliths are observed outside the pelvis, intestinal hemangiomas should be suspected (less likely, calcified parasitic cysts).

Nonvascular calcifications include opaque medications (i.e., iron and calcium pills), calculi (gallbladder, urinary tract, and appendicoliths), dystrophic calcifications (inflammatory lesions such as calcified mesenteric nodes or calcified granulomas in the liver and/or spleen), calcifications from developmental lesions such as dermoids and teratomas, and, finally, neoplastic calcifications, such as mucin-secreting adenocarcinomas.

Metastasis can produce faint calcification within the abdominal cavity, particularly in the area of the liver, the peritoneal surfaces of an organ, the wall of the bowel, and around the pelvis.

To summarize, in following this systematic approach you should start with the "least important" structures (such as those observed in the four corners of a 14×17 cm abdominal roentgenogram), the fat-muscle interfaces (particularly in the flanks, the iliopsoas regions, the obturator internus, and the periformis muscles), then proceed to the hollow viscus, and, finally, to the solid organs of the alimentary and genitourinary tracts.

In addition to faulty interpretation of the radiological findings and technical errors, the lack of an appropriate clinical history may result in improper interpretation of findings, and so a thorough knowledge of the patient's history is essential before any type of radiological examination. Needless to say, contrast studies of the abdominal organs may result in complications due to wrong indications (clinical condition of the patient), improper performance of the radiological examination, reactions to contrast media or medications, or from the instrumentation utilized.

In this book we shall consider (a) the liver, spleen, and pancreas, and (b), the hollow viscera of the alimentary tract.

Atlas

Figures 1–50

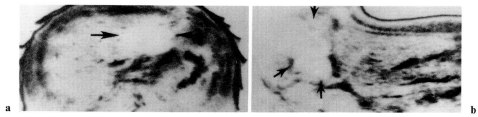

Fig. 1 a, b. Heart motion causing hypoechoic areas in the left lobe of the liver. Axial (**a**) and sagittal (**b**) echographic studies of the liver. Note hypoechoic area in topography of the left lobe simulating a cystic mass. This was the result of the contraction of the heart and transmitted pulsations to the left lobe of the liver. The use of proper echographic technique and changes of position ot the patient may cause this pseudoabnormality to disappear

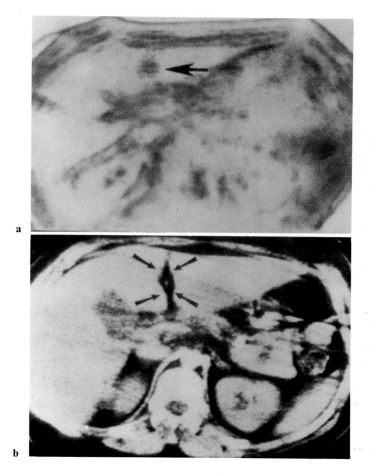

Fig. 2a, b. Ligamentum teres simulating hepatic mass. **a** US examination shows a focal hyperechoic area in the left lobe of the liver. **b** CT shows the classic features of the ligamentum teres. Occasionally, abundance of fat will cause focal echogenicity on ultrasound examination and low CT values in the topography of the ligamentum teres

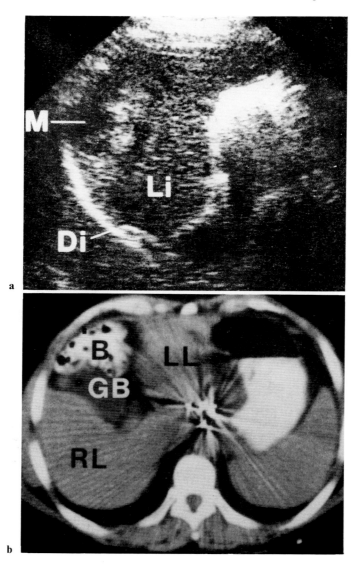

Fig. 3a, b. Interposition of the bowel. **a** US examination shows an apparent mass (*M*) under the diaphragm (*DI*); *LI* liver. **b** Computed tomographic examination of the same patient. Note that the opacified bowel (*B*) with the gallbladder (*GB*) behind is interposed between the right lobe (*RL*) and the left lobe (*LL*) of the liver. Occasionally, on chest or abdominal radiography, one may see a radiolucency under the right dome of the diaphragm which is neither free air nor fat but air in the bowel interposed between the liver and the right dome of the diaphragm (Chilaiditi syndrome)

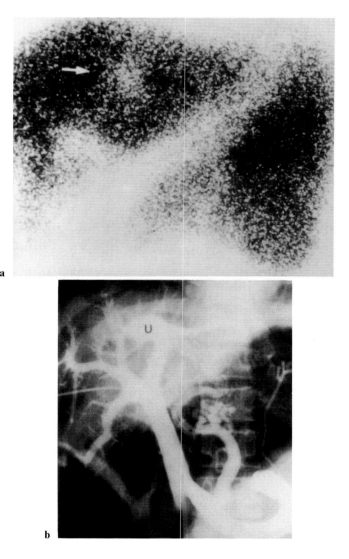

Fig. 4a, b. Dilated umbilical vein simulating focal hepatic mass. **a** Phagocytic liver scan reveals a photopenic area in the center of the liver (*arrow*). **b** Transhepatic portogram. A dilated umbilical vein (*U*), secondary to portal hypertension, and enlarged tributaries of the portal vein are observed. The umbilical vein(s) can enlarge as an anterior collateral pathway in patients with portal hypertension. By sonography, scintigraphy, and CT they can simulate a liver mass. Duplex sonographic study provides pathognomonic information as to the cause of this focal mass

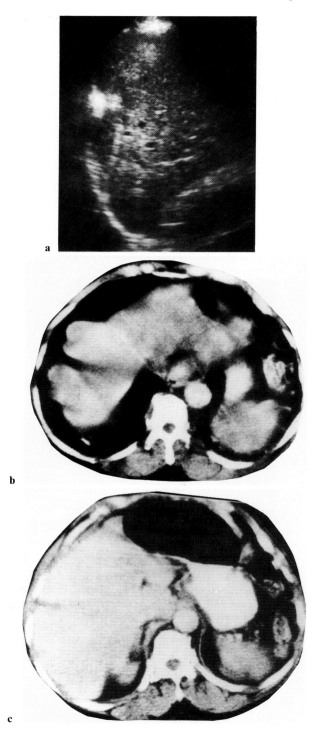

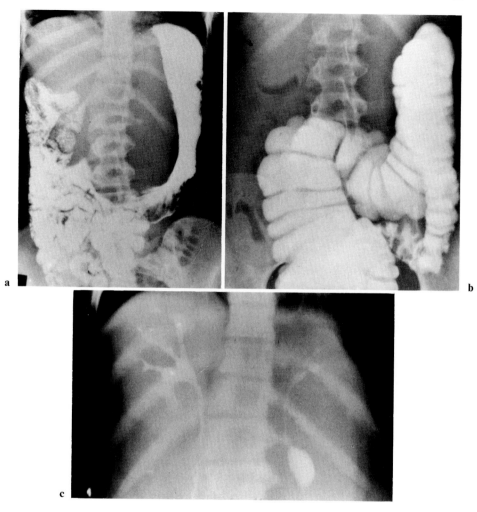

Fig. 6a–c. A dysplastic liver secondary to omphalocele. **a** Upper GI series and **b** barium enema of a patient who presented with an asymptomatic large epigastric mass. Note the compression and displacement of the stomach and the high position of the small bowel suggesting an enlarged left lobe of the liver and a small right lobe. The barium enema shows a medial position of the ascending colon. **c** Representative film of an intravenous urogram. Note the subdiaphragmatic position of the right kidney with a prominent upper pole. The left kidney also appears in a subdiaphragmatic position and is hypoplastic. A diverticulum of the left ureter is present. (From Margulis and Burhenne 1973)

Fig. 5a–c. Accessory hepatic fissure(s) simulating hepatic mass. **a** Sonographic examination of the liver showing what appears to be a mass in the right subdiaphragmatic region. **b, c** reveal the accessory hepatic fissure which often contains diaphragmatic muscle indenting the right lobe of the liver

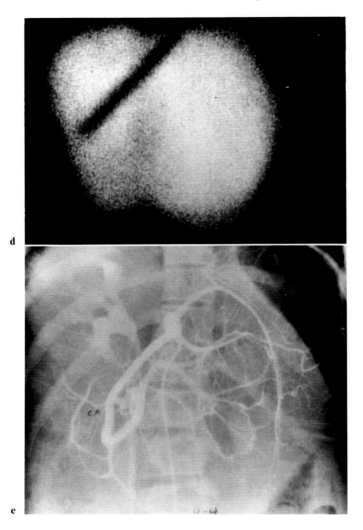

Fig. 6d–g. A dysplastic liver secondary to omphalocele. **d** A phagocytic liver scan. Note the uniform enlargement of the left lobe of the liver without evidence of focal defect. A rib marker accounts for the oblique band running across the liver. **e** A selective celiac arteriogram showing inversion of the celiac trunk. There are prominent branches of the hepatic artery without signs of neovascularity. **f** Late phase of celiac artery injection showing uniform opacification of the liver without evidence of a mass. **g** Selective left renal arteriogram. Note the dysplastic left kidney and the enlarged left adrenal gland. The patient had multiple anomalies resulting from an omphalocele that was corrected shortly after birth. The liver developed in the hernial sac and when repositioned into the abdominal cavity was already dysplastic. The two kidneys ascended to the subdiaphragmatic region. There were also anomalies of the left urinary tract and of the left adrenal gland. The "mass" was the result of an intrinsically normal large left lobe of the liver; the right lobe was hypoplastic. (From Margulis and Burhenne 1973)

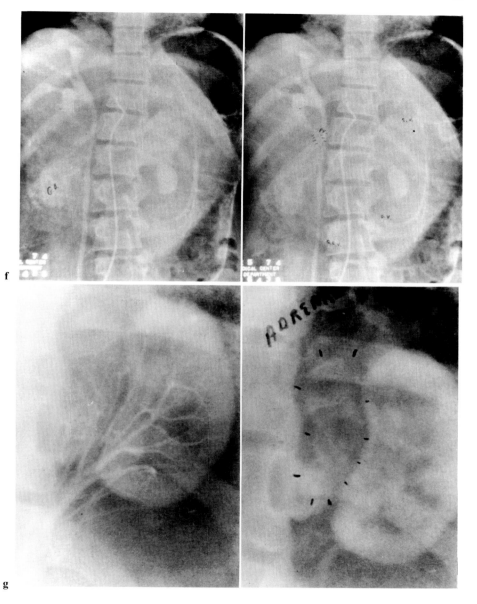

f

g

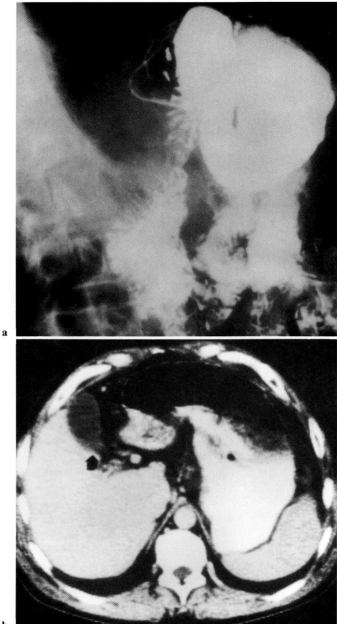

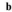

Fig. 7a, b. Congenital absence of the left lobe of the liver producing an abnormal position of the small bowel following partial gastrectomy. The patient had a Billroth II procedure. **a** Following surgery a control examination revealed an abnormally high position of the small bowel. Adhesions, technical error, and a gastric volvulus were considered. **b** CT examination reveals the absence of the left lobe of the liver. *Arrow* points to a normal gallbladder. The absence of liver tissue allowed the bowel to ascend to a subdiaphragmatic position

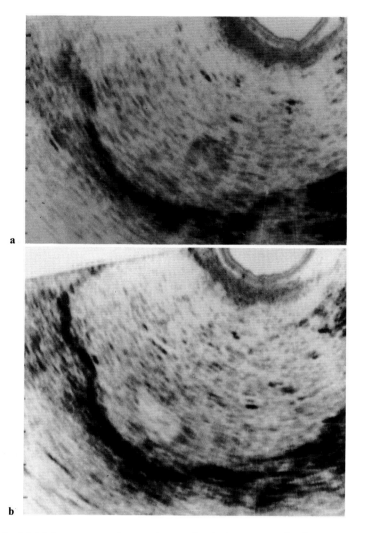

a

b

Fig. 8 a, b. Multiple cavernous hemangiomas simulating metastatic disease. A 67-year-old man presented with considerable weight loss and jaundice. US examination (**a** and **b**) revealed multiple focal abnormalities characterized by increased echogenicity and hypoechoic and complex lesions

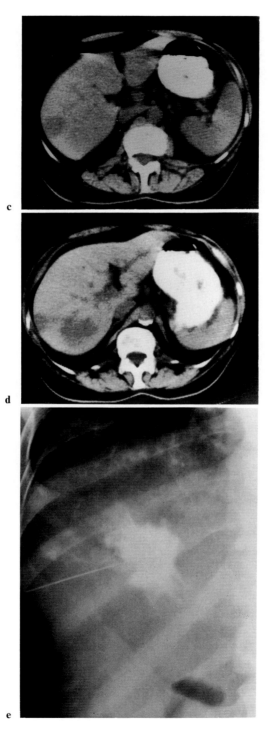

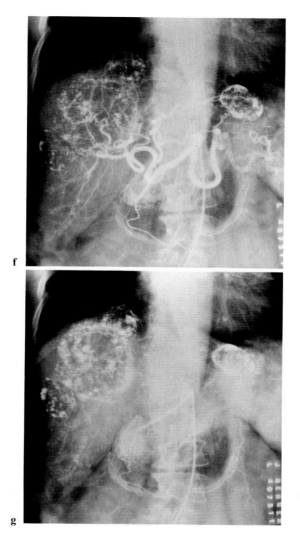

Fig. 8c–g. Multiple cavernous hemangiomas simulating metastatic disease. CT of the liver (**c** and **d**) revealed multiple low density masses scattered through the liver. Needle biopsy under CT guidance (**e**) was performed and blood was retrieved. Cytologic and histologic examination failed to diagnose the cause of the mass. Contrast medium was injected and dispersed irregularly in the cavity. Extensive clinical and radiological examination of this patient failed to reveal a primary tumor. Laparoscopy or mini-laparatomy was advised to attain a definitive diagnosis; the patient refused. Instead he sold his properties, valued at millions of dollars, divorced his wife and married a young woman, and took a cruise around the world. After a 3-month vacation, he returned to Miami, free of jaundice, with a 20 pound weight gain and feeling great! The patient agreed to a celiac examination. The celiac arteriogram (**f** and **g**) revealed multiple hypervascular masses with the characteristic appearance of cavernous hemangiomas. Note that the feeding arteries are not enlarged; there is no evidence of venous obstruction nor arteriovenous communications. Typical rim opacification and prolonged retention of contrast in these masses were observed; all are characteristic features of cavernous hemangiomas. Retrospectively, the patient had a viral hepatitis but no tumor. Although his self-management strategy proved beneficial, I cannot recommend it to anyone!

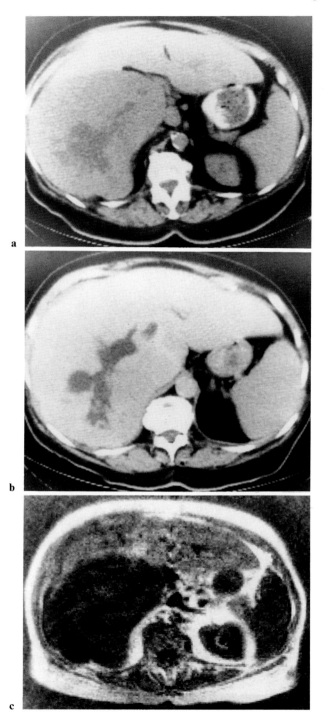

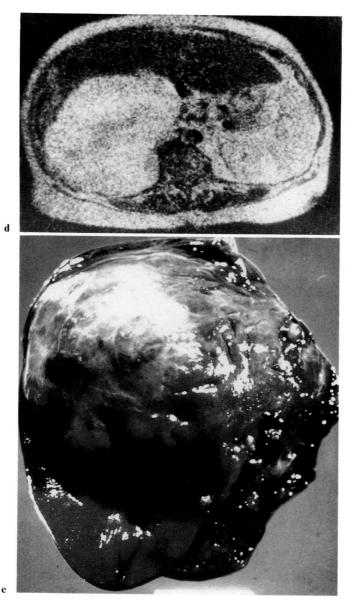

Fig. 9a–e. Another example of cavernous hemangioma studied by **a, b** CT and **c, d** by MRI. The CT study shows a hypodense area with irregular lucencies primarily in the center of the mass. A late phase of the enhanced CT examination (**b**) reveals uniform opacification of most of the mass except for its center which remains radiolucent. A T1-weighted MR image (**c**) shows low signal intensity at the level of the well-circumscribed mass. The T2-weighted image (**d**) shows a hyperintense mass with a slight heterogeneous appearance and a well-demarcated outline. The CT and MR appearances are not pathognomonic. Occasionally, hepatomas, particularly fibrolamellar hepatoma, focal nodular hyperplasia, and other lesions can show a rounded configuration with a center of different density. Hypersignal in the MR image may be related to blood or to the hypervascularity of a central scar (i.e., nodular hyperplasia). **e** Gross examination of a cavernous hemangioma. The lesion is reddish and the uncut specimen resembles a hepatoma

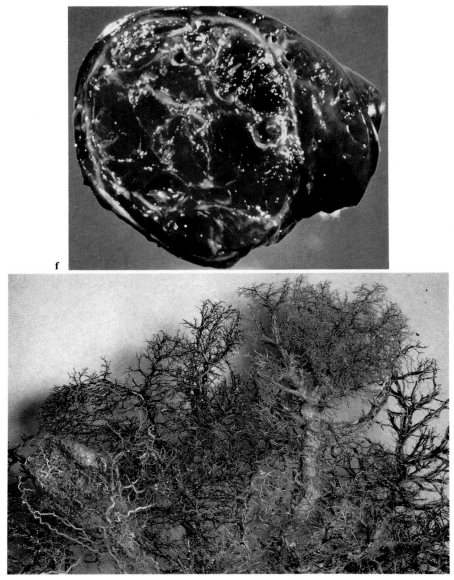

Fig. 9 f, g. f Another example of cavernous hemangioma. The cut section of the tumor shows hemorrhagic areas. Note dark blood clots and numerous septa. This morphology explains the variability of the echographic findings and the anatomical basis for the CT and MR findings. **g** A cast-corrosion preparation showing the arterial hypervascularity of several cavernous hemangiomas

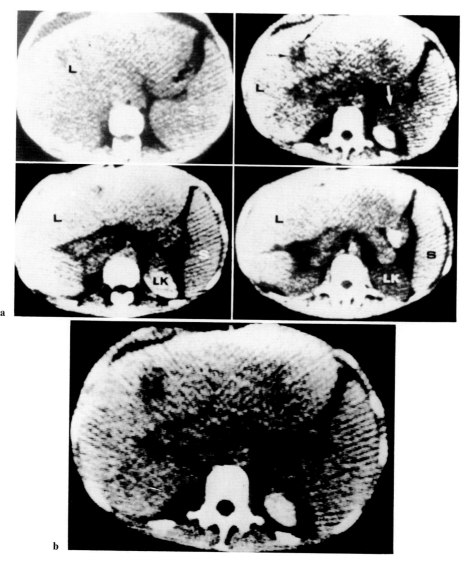

Fig. 10 a, b. Zand infarcts. A 43-year-old woman who, while traveling through Mexico with her husband and two children, noted a prominent abdomen. On palpation of her abdomen, her husband, who is a surgeon, suspected hepatomegaly. She had no history of diarrhea, abdominal pain, or any type of general symptoms. **a** Upon return to Miami he ordered a CT examination that revealed hepatosplenomegaly, focal low density areas in the liver (*arrows*), and a mass in topography of the hilus of the spleen (*white arrow*). **b** A representative CT section obtained with an old CT machine showed low density areas in the liver and evidence of hepatosplenomegaly. (From Margulis and Burhenne 1973)

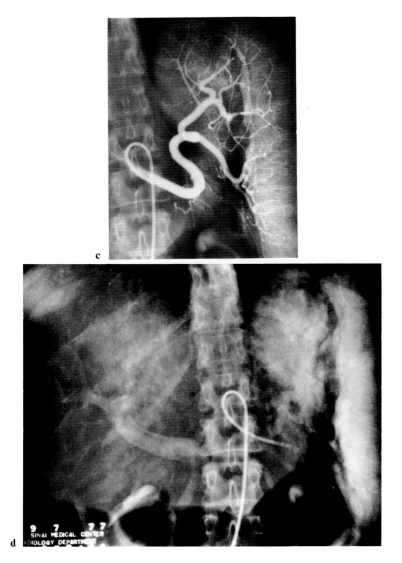

c

d

Fig. 10c–g. Zand infarcts. An arteriogram was ordered. **c** Selective splenic artery injection showed diffuse hepatosplenomegaly, no evidence of intrinsic involvement of the splenic artery, no evidence of neovascularity in topography of the body and tail of the pancreas. **d** A venous phase of the selective splenic artery injection. Note complete occlusion of the splenic vein and numerous, enlarged veins in topography of the splenic hilus (collateral circulation). This latter finding explained the mass seen on the CT examination. The left branch of the portal vein was not visualized. (From Margulis and Burhenne 1973)

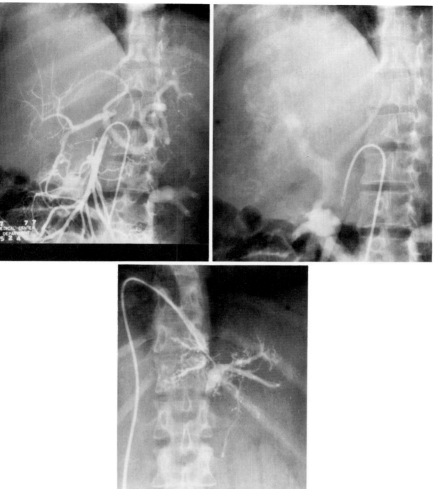

e–g. Selective superior mesenteric arteriogram (**e**) revealed reflux of contrast into the hepatic artery. No evidence of neovascularity was noted in the liver. The venous phase of the superior mesenteric artery injection (**f**) showed absent opacification of the left branch of the portal vein. Initially the diagnosis entertained was that of a tumor of the tail of the pancreas, obstructing the splenic vein and causing splenomegaly and liver metastases. The second diagnosis considered was that of lymphoma. The surgeon was firm in his impression that his wife had no evidence of malignancy. Following the CT and angiographic examinations another tentative diagnosis was that of hepatoma. However, contradicting the diagnosis of a hepatoma was the absence of neovascularity and that the splenic vein was obstructed but not the main portal vein. **g** We suggested hepatic venography which was then performed. Note obstruction of hepatic veins with numerous intrahepatic, intra- and intervenous collaterals. This appearance is classic for veno-occlusive disease. (From Margulis and Burhenne 1973)

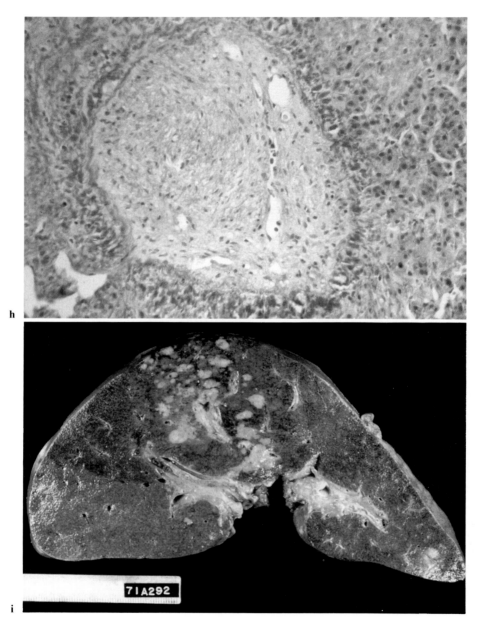

Fig. 10h, i. Zand infarcts. **h** A needle biopsy revealed occlusion of central hepatic venules with numerous small veins representing intrahepatic collateral circulation. Fibrosis of central hepatic lobules and congestive changes without signs of cirrhosis or of tumor were reported. The patient eventually died. **i** The liver showed multiple yellow nodules suggesting metastasis. However, these actually represent Zand infarcts (liver infarcts secondary to occlusion of hepatic veins). Table 1 (Appendix) lists some causes of veno-occlusive disease. Of all possible etiologies this woman gave a history of being an habitual tea drinker. In certain parts of the world, like Jamaica, there are tea leaves which contain a high concentration of *Senecio* alkaloid. This chemical is known to cause veno-occlusive disease. We assumed that this was the cause of this syndrome of veno-occlusive disease

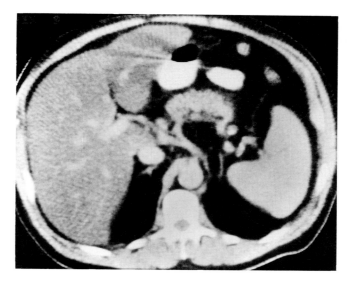

Fig. 11. Diffuse fatty infiltration causing diffuse hepatomegaly. The patient was receiving hyperalimentation. CT scan shows the diffuse low density area of the liver with conspicuous branches of the portal vein. Note that the liver is less dense than the spleen. Biopsy: fatty metamorphosis. For further details see Fig. 13

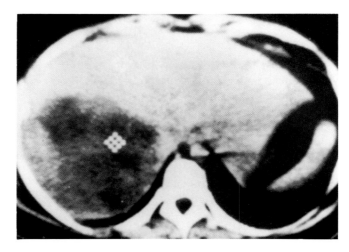

Fig. 12. A focal hepatic mass in the right lobe of the liver simulating a liver tumor. The CT appearance mimics a primary or metastatic tumor of the liver. At biopsy this was found to be focal fatty metamorphosis. For further details see Fig. 13

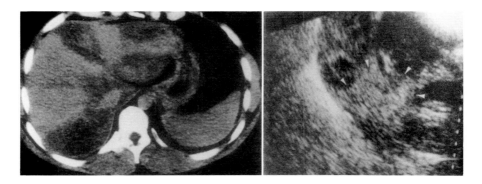

Fig. 13. Multiple fatty masses. Patient had an abnormal biochemical profile suggesting liver disease. The CT examination (*left*) shows multiple triangular low density areas. Differential diagnosis would have to include fatty masses, liver infarcts, and liver tumors. US examination (*right*) showed speckled echogenicity. This suggests the presence of fat, which was confirmed on liver biopsy. The echographic appearance of fat in the liver can vary from single, multiple, or diffuse echographic abnormalities. The lesions can be hyperechoic, hypoechoic, or have mixed echogenicity. A clue to the diagnosis of a fatty liver mass is to demonstrate nonenlarged vessels crossing the mass. Causes of fatty liver are listed in Table 2 (Appendix). Note that intravenous hyperalimentation and high doses of steroid therapy are two iatrogenic causes of fatty metamorphosis of the liver. When a patient with cancer presents with hepatomegaly, the enlarged liver may not be related to a malignancy but to fatty metamorphosis induced by the treatment

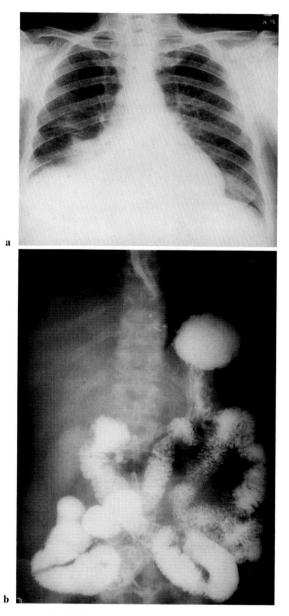

a

b

Fig. 14 a, b. Sarcoma of the IVC. A 36-year-old teacher presented with chest pain, hemo-
physis, and ascites. **a** Frontal chest roentgenogram. Note the right middle lobe infiltrate,
reduced volume of the right lower lobe, and fluid in the right costodiaphragmatic angle and
right minor fissure. Note the high position of the diaphragm and diffuse density below the
diaphragm suggesting ascites and/or organomegaly. **b** Upper GI series. Diffuse enlargement
of the liver was observed. No intrinsic lesion of the upper alimentary tract was noted. There
was no evidence of portal hypertension (no signs of varices)

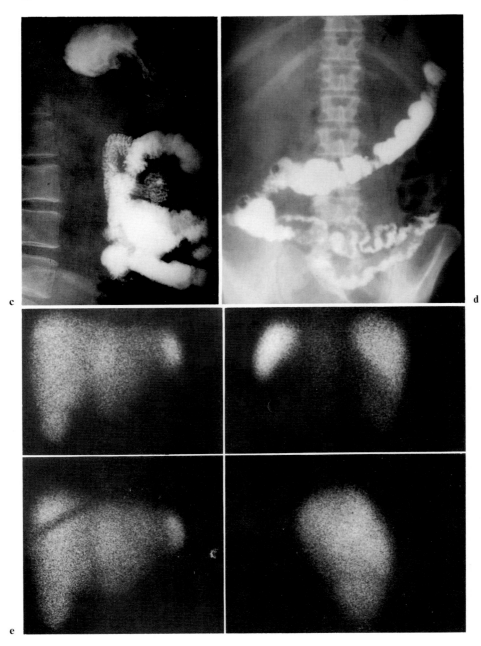

c   d

e

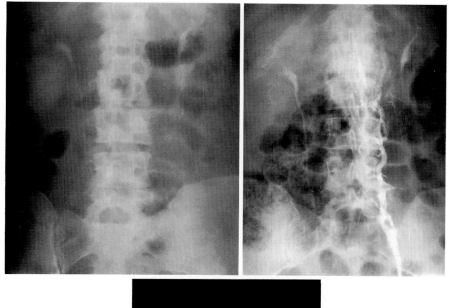

f   g

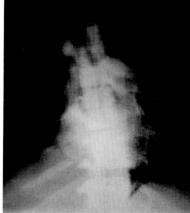

h

Fig. 14c–h. Sarcoma of the IVC. **c** Upper GI series providing the clue to the diagnosis. Note anterior displacement of the second part of the duodenum. This finding is usually the result of a pancreatic mass, an enlarged abdominal aorta, adenopathies, or a retroperitoneal tumor. **d** Postevacuation film of a barium enema. Note diffuse displacement of the colon. No intrinsic lesion of the bowel was observed. **e** Phagocytic scan. Diffuse hepatomegaly without focal lesions of the liver was noted. There was no evidence of splenomegaly. **f** Intravenous urogram showing the kidneys normal in size, shape, and position, with good excretion of the contrast medium bilaterally. Discrete notching was noted along the ureters. **g** An attempt to study the inferior vena cava. The left femoral vein was injected. Total obstruction of the left iliac vein and inferior vena cava was present with collateral circulation to the perivertebral venous plexus and to the ascending lumbar veins. **h** A repeat injection of the left femoral vein shows absent opacification of the inferior vena cava. Note a markedly enlarged azygos vein. A density was noted in the right cardiodiaphragmatic angle, intially interpreted as representing pericardial effusion. This density proved to represent an enlarged inferior vena cava

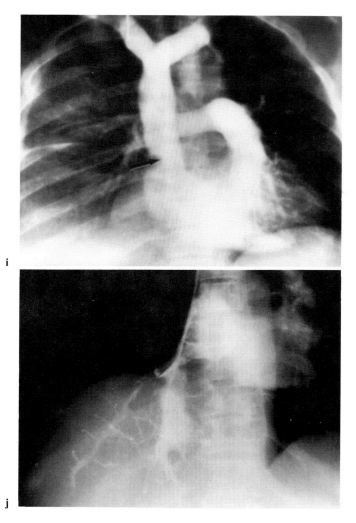

Fig. 14i–l. Sarcoma of the IVC. **i** Angiocardiogram, dextro phase. Note filling defect in the right atrium (*arrow*). The density to the right of the right atrium is not related to the heart or pericardium but to a markedly enlarged inferior vena cava. **j** A catheter was advanced into the right atrium and then into the terminal portion of the inferior vena cava. The catheter could not be advanced beyond the distal inferior vena cava. Contrast material was injected at that level and revealed obstruction of the hepatic veins and of the inferior vena cava and a mass in the right atrium. **k** Selective celiac arteriogram. Note neovascularity at the level of the liver with shunting of the contrast medium into the hepatic veins. This study was interpreted as demonstrating a hypervascular liver mass compatible with a hepatoma. **l** Late phase of selective celiac injection. Note neovascularity in the center of the liver with filling of hepatic veins. The distribution of the abnormal vessels should have suggested the mass to represent a tumor of the inferior vena cava rather than a tumor of the liver

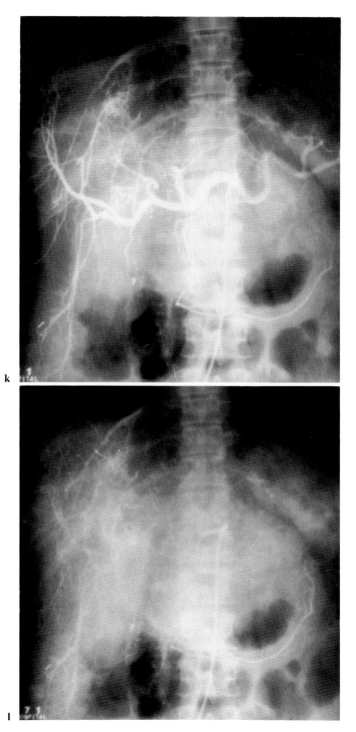

k

l

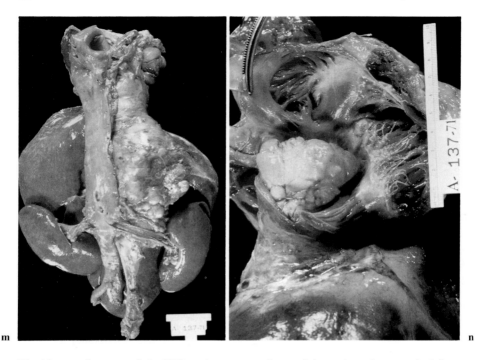

Fig. 14 m–p. Sarcoma of the IVC. **m** Autopsy specimen of the patient photographed from behind (dorsal view). Note the massively enlarged inferior vena cava which was a solid structure. There was occlusion of the two renal veins. **n** A ventral view of the right side of the heart opened. Note mass protruding into the right atrium. This was a tumor of the inferior vena cava growing into the right atrium. Below the tumor one can see the massively enlarged inferior vena cava (which simulated a pericardial process). **o** Histologic section. Note that the lumen of the inferior vena cava is filled by tumor (leiomyosarcoma). Note also the hypervascular wall of the inferior vena cava. It represents the expanded vasa vasorum supplied by the celiac artery. This explains the neovascularity noted on the celiac arteriogram. **p** Late phase of the celiac arteriogram. Note that the blush corresponds to the hepatic segment of the inferior vena cava. This patient had a pseudoneoplasia of the liver due to a leiomyosarcoma of the inferior vena cava causing obstruction of the hepatic veins and hepatomegaly

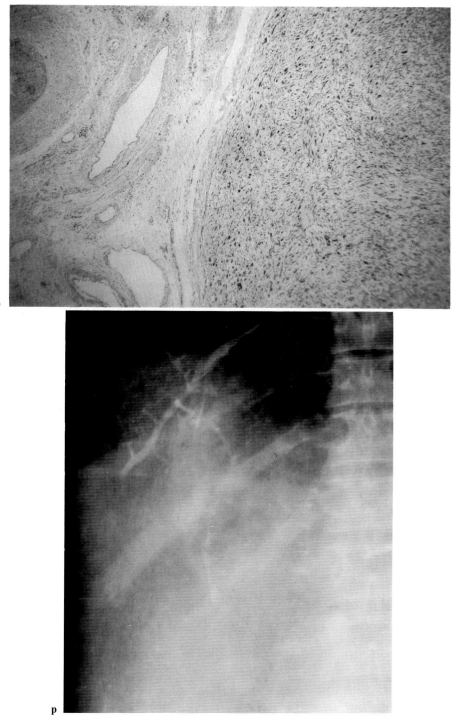

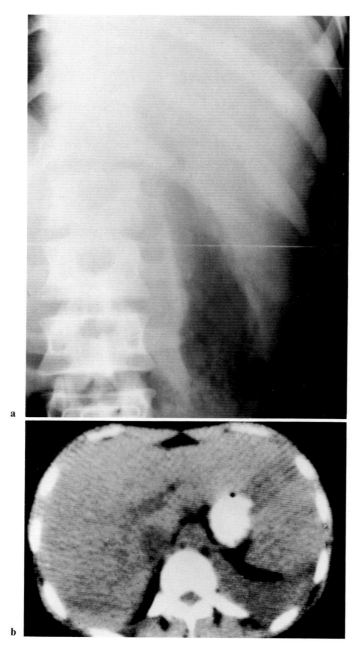

Fig. 15a, b. Pseudosplenomegaly. This patient had a history of alcoholic liver disease. **a** Scout film of the abdomen showed the stomach displaced medially and downward by apparent splenomegaly. **b** CT of the abdomen with contrast in the stomach. Note the marked hepatomegaly. The left lobe of the liver reached the left flank and was the cause of the dorsal and medial displacement of the stomach

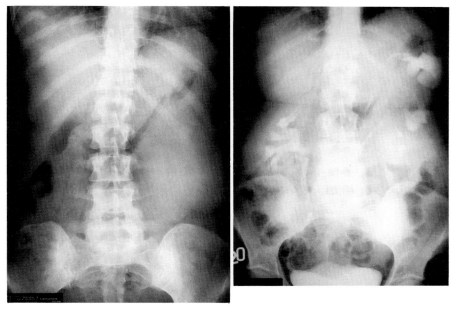

Fig. 16 a, b. A 40-year-old woman with anemia of unexplained etiology, hepatomegaly, and "splenomegaly." **a** Frontal view of the abdomen revealed prominence of the liver shadow and superior and medial displacement of the stomach. A mass was palpable under the left rib cage and suggested an enlarged spleen. The working diagnosis was a lymphoproliferative disorder. Bone marrow study and a splenic pulp aspiration did not reveal the cause of the anemia. An extensive workup was undertaken that included an upper and lower GI series. A liver scan showed diffuse hepatomegaly. Liver biopsy failed to reveal evidence of metastatic disease. At this time no definitive diagnosis was made. **b** An intravenous urogram was ordered and an enlarged left kidney with a duplicated collecting system was noted. Carcinoma of the left kidney was immediately suspected and an arteriogram was ordered.

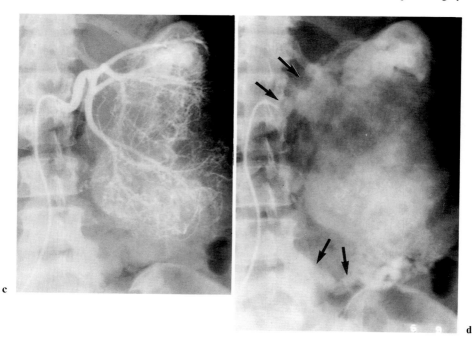

c

d

Fig. 16 c–f. A 40-year-old woman with anemia of unexplained etiology, hepatomegaly, and "splenomegaly." **c** A selective left renal arteriogram. Note a huge tumor of the left kidney with abundant neovascularity. **d** Venous phase of the study. The left renal vein never opacified. Extensive collateral venous circulation (*arrows*) was noted. There were left adrenal and lymph node metastases. **e** A celiac arteriogram showed a cephalically displaced, nonenlarged spleen (*S*). The renal mass (*M*) was the cause of the left upper quadrant mass. Selective celiac arteriogram (not shown) revealed stretched hepatic arteries but no evidence of neovascularity. **f** The patient had surgery and a very large renal carcinoma was confirmed. The hepatomegaly was not related to metastatic disease but to the "hepatic dysfunction syndrome" observed in about 10% of patients with renal cell carcinoma. It must be remembered that renal cell carcinoma can be clinically silent (no flank pain, palpable mass, or hematuria) in about 20% of patients. Hepatomegaly and/or liver function tests may return to normal following the resection of the tumor. In this patient the hepatic dysfunction was secondary to the presence of a renal cell carcinoma. Likewise in a patient with splenomegaly of unknown cause, one should look for a malignant melanoma. When the malignant melanoma is removed the spleen may return to a normal size. Table 3 (Appendix) lists the systemic effects of renal cell carcinoma

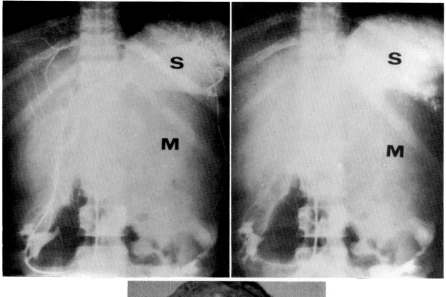

e

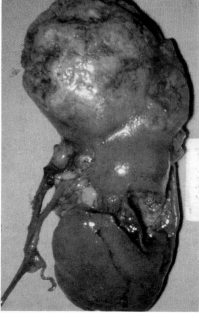

f

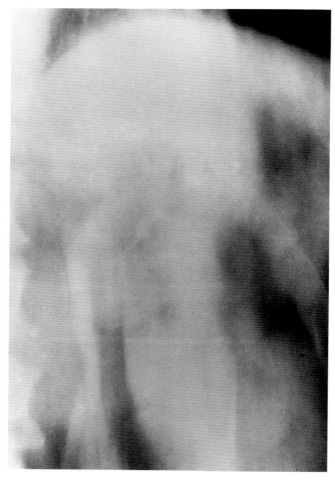

a

Fig. 17a–d. Wandering spleen simulating splenomegaly. An asymptomatic 50-year-old man had a palpable mass in the left upper quadrant. Clinically the diagnosis was splenomegaly. **a** Tomogram of an intravenous urogram. Note a subdiaphragmatic left kidney and a mass projecting below the left kidney. The impression was that of a renal cyst or a predunculated renal tumor. That the shadow of the spleen was not seen in its usual location (in the subdiaphragmatic region of the left upper quadrant) was not appreciated. **b** Selective left renal arteriogram revealed a subdiaphragmatic normal left kidney. Note the wide dimensions of this kidney. No intrinsic abnormality of the left kidney was present. **c** Selective splenic arteriogram shows that the mass below the left kidney was a nonenlarged spleen. The spleen is not in its usual location. This is an anomaly related to the absence of the normal splenic attachments such as the phrenicocolic ligament. **d** Phagocytic scan. (From Margulis and Burhenne 1973).

Note the spleen in an abnormally low position. Noninvasive imaging modalities such as ultrasonography, scintigraphy, computed tomography, and magnetic resonance imaging can be used to recognize the presence of a wandering spleen.

Wandering spleens can simulate splenomegaly or any other type of abdominal mass. The hypermobility of the spleen predisposes this organ to thrombosis of the splenic vein from a twist of the splenic pedicle. This has been particularly reported during pregnancy

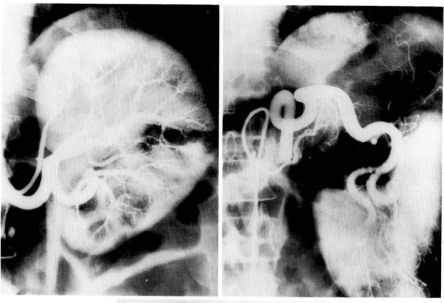

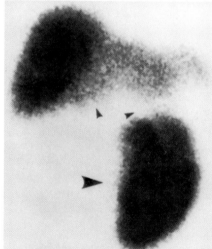

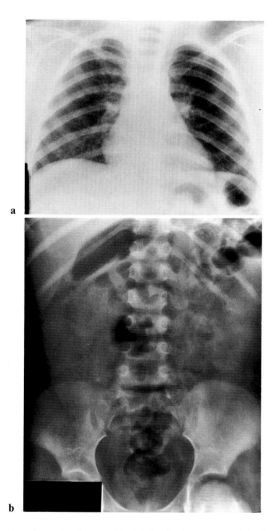

Fig. 18a–g. Ectopic spleen. An 8-year-old child had a history of a left diaphragmatic hernia, repaired shortly after birth. The child presented with a mass in the right flank. **a** Frontal view of the chest. Note slight decrease in the left pulmonary markings and a normal position of the diaphragm. This is probably the result of an expanded hypoplastic left lung. **b** Supine view of the abdomen. A mass is noted in the right flank. It was initially interpreted as a prominent right lobe of the liver. The stomach appeared in an unusual position (slightly to the right of the midline). **c** Intravenous urogram revealed the kidneys normal in size, shape, and position. Note that the right flank mass does not appear to be related to the liver or to the kidney. The stomach is again noted to be in the right upper quadrant. **d** Upper GI series. This study confirms the stomach to be abnormal in position, with the bowel in the left upper quadrant and no evidence of a splenic shadow. **e** A barium enema showed the large bowel malrotated. The cecum and ascending colon are not in their usual location (right iliac fossa). Note that the shadow of the spleen is not visualized. **f** Frontal view and **g** lateral view of a phagocytic scan. Note the liver in a normal location and with a normal appearance. Below the liver is the spleen, which appears intrinsically normal but with an abnormal shape. Splenic ectopia was the cause of the right flank mass. (Courtesy of Dr. A. Y. de Paula Lobo, Recife, Brazil)

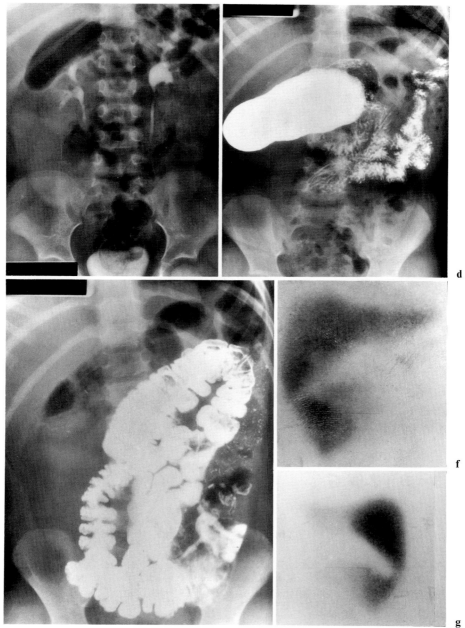

c
d
e
f
g

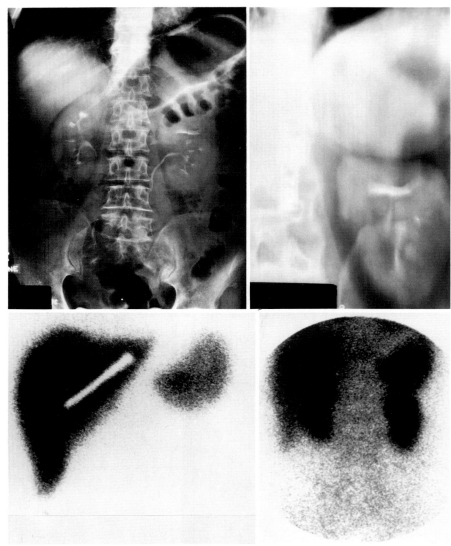

a

b

c

d

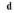

Fig. 19a–d. Malrotation of the spleen. A 60-year-old patient reported urinary frequency. An intravenous urogram was ordered. **a** Early phase of the study. Note flattening of the left upper calyces with the suggestion of a left suprarenal mass. **b** A tomogram showing the superior concavity of the upper pole of the left kidney, flattening of the left upper calyces, and a rounded left suprarenal mass. **c** Phagocytic scan. Note a malrotated normal-sized spleen. Its inferior margin is convex. **d** Superimposed phagocytic and renal scan. Note the contiguity of the spleen to the left kidney. The upper pole of the left kidney was not convex due to the malrotated spleen that produced a compression of the upper pole of the left kidney and simulated an adrenal mass or a pancreatic tumor

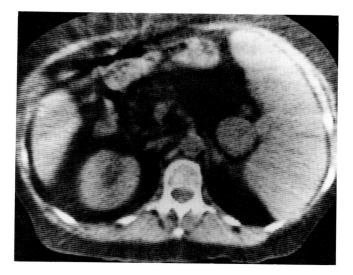

Fig. 20. An asymptomatic accessory spleen in a patient presenting with splenomegaly. CT of the abdomen shows an enlarged spleen and a rounded mass in the topography of the splenic hilus. This mass might be confused with an adrenal tumor, an adenopathy, or a pancreatic neoplasm. It represents an accessory spleen. The left adrenal gland and the pancreas were normal. (From Margulis and Burhenne 1973)

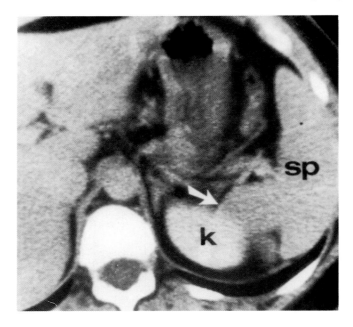

Fig. 21. Heterotopic spleen simulating left renal mass. A CT examination of this patient showed splenic tissue projecting ventral to the left kidney and in anatomic proximity. Initially a left renal tumor was suspected. An enhanced CT examination revealed the mass to be unrelated to the left kidney. *K*, left kidney; *SP*, spleen; *arrow*, mass

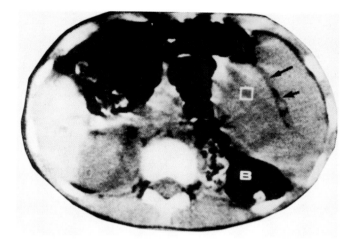

Fig. 22. Heterotopic spleen simulating a tumor in the left upper quadrant. A CT examination shows a mass medial to the spleen. Its posterior aspect is in direct continuity with the dorsal portion of the spleen. This is an anatomic variant which produces the appearance of a bilobed spleen

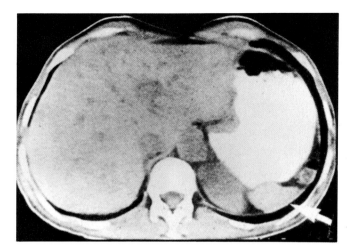

Fig. 23. A mass (*arrow*) behind the stomach in a patient who had a splenectomy. This mass corresponds to a splenic remnant and should not be confused with a tumor. Occasionally, following surgery, portions of splenic tissue can remain in the abdomen or seed the pleural cavities simulating different types of tumors. Scintigraphic examination or CT are quite useful to recognize residual splenic tissue in the abdominal or pleural cavities

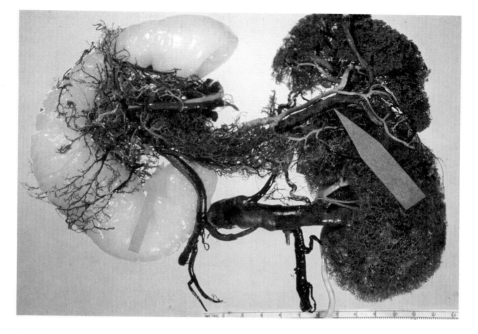

Fig. 24. A cast-corrosion study of the duodenum, pancreas, spleen, left adrenal gland, and left kidney. Note the head of the pancreas surrounded by the duodenum. The *right arrow* points to the superior mesenteric vein. The *left arrow head* points to the splenic vein. Note the anatomic proximity of the tail of the pancreas to the hilus of the spleen, to the upper pole of the left kidney, and to the left adrenal gland. Note also proximity of the left renal vein and left adrenal veins to the pancreas. Intervenous anastomoses normally are observed between the spleen, the upper pole of the left kidney, the tail of the pancreas, and the left adrenal gland

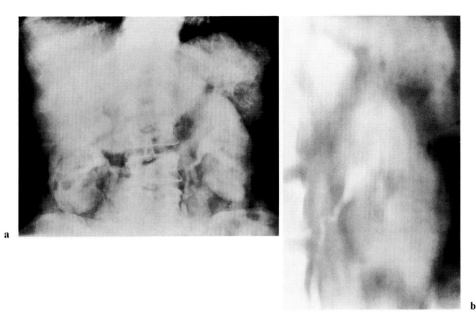

a

b

Fig. 25 a–e. Normal dorsally directed tail of the pancreas. A patient presented with urinary frequency and dysuria. An intravenous urogram was ordered. **a** There is a mass close to the upper pole of the left kidney. **b** Tomogram from the urographic examination. The mass appears to be separate from the upper pole of the left kidney. An adrenal tumor was considered, although the mass is somewhat high for it to be the left adrenal gland. **c** Selective celiac arteriogram. Note that in the arterial phase (*top*) there is no neovascularity and in the venous phase (*bottom*) a hyperintense tail of the pancreas (*P*) is visualized. The patient had no evidence of a pancreatic disorder. Neither an islet cell tumor nor any other type of pancreatic neoplasm was present. **d** CT studies (*top* and *bottom*). Note the dorsally directed tail of the pancreas. Seen on end, it simulated a tumor projected above the upper pole of the left kidney. The left adrenal gland was normal. **e** Scintigraphic examination (dorsal view). Note simultaneous scanning of the liver and of the pancreas. The rounded hyperintense area to the left of the liver represents the tail of the pancreas seen on end

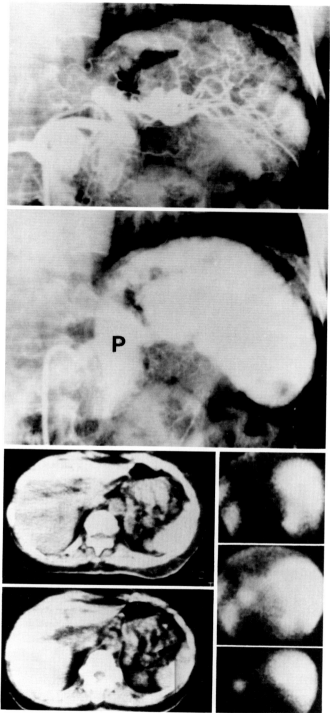

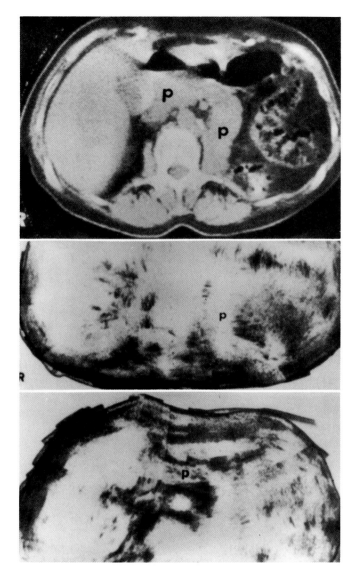

Fig. 26. Relocated tail of the pancreas following left nephrectomy. A density was noted in the left upper quadrant of uncertain etiology. A CT examination (*top*) shows a dorsally directed tail of the pancreas (*P*). Ultrasound examination (*middle* and *bottom*) revealed a normal pancreas. This patient had a relocated pancreatic tail which occupied the space vacated by the left kidney. Also, the bowel tends to partially fill the renal fossa following left nephrectomy

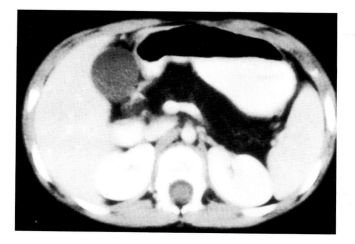

Fig. 27. CT of a patient with abundant peripancreatic fat. Obesity, Cushing's syndrome, and cystic fibrosis are among the most common causes of peripancreatic fat accumulation. The pancreas is often replaced by fat in elderly patients

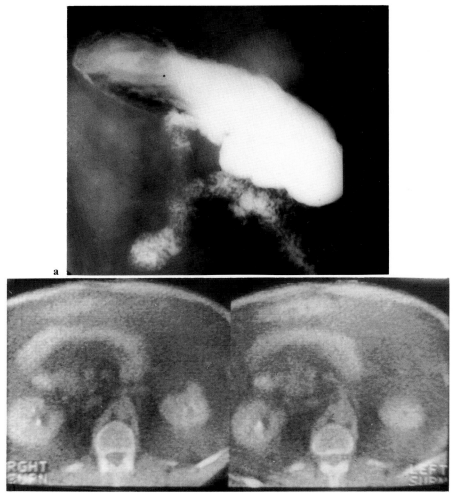

Fig. 28 a, b. Retroduodenal adiposity simulating a pancreatic mass. This very obese patient presented with nonspecific abdominal pain. **a** A lateral view of an upper GI series revealed anterior displacement of the second part of the duodenum. A pancreatic tumor, adenopathy, and an aneurysm of the aorta were considered. **b** A CT scan revealed excessive fat and no evidence of a tumor

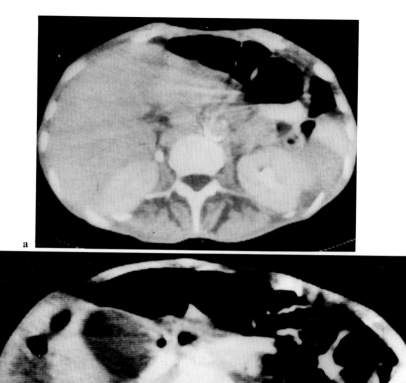

Fig. 29 a, b. A patient who had experienced extreme weight loss. **a** CT of the abdomen. Note densities surrounding the abdominal aorta. They were interpreted as probable adenopathies or a retroperitoneal tumor. **b** A CT section at another level showed a distended gallbladder. Note in both **a** and **b** the absence of subcutaneous fat. This patient was explored and no tumor was found.

Absence of fat in the retroperitoneum can simulate a tumor by coalescence of bowel loops. Their proximity to the abdominal aorta can simulate adenopathies in nonenhanced CT examinations. The small bowel should always be identifiable on abdominal CT or MR examinations in order to differentiate loops of bowel from extraintestinal masses

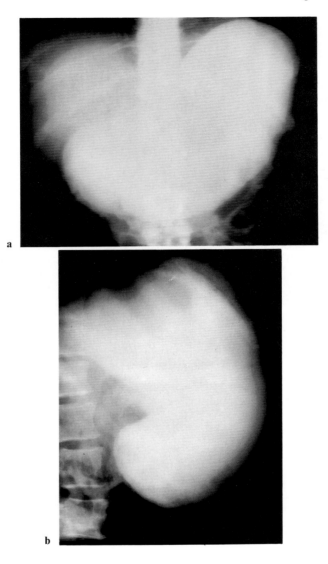

Fig. 30 a–d. Injected pancreatic pseudocyst simulating gastric dilatation, **a, b** The opacified structure has the appearance of a stomach; **c** opacified bowel loops. **d** Air was introduced through a tube in the stomach. The opacified structure was retrogastric and corresponded to a pancreatic pseudocyst which had been injected with contrast material. Clinical history is mandatory for the correct interpretation of radiographic abnormalities

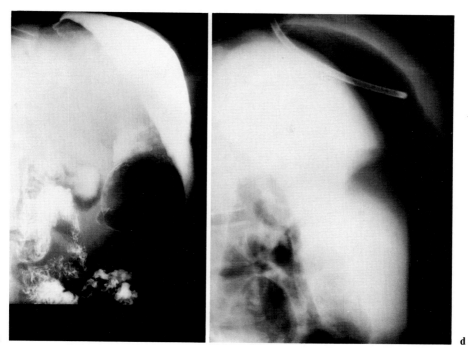

c   d

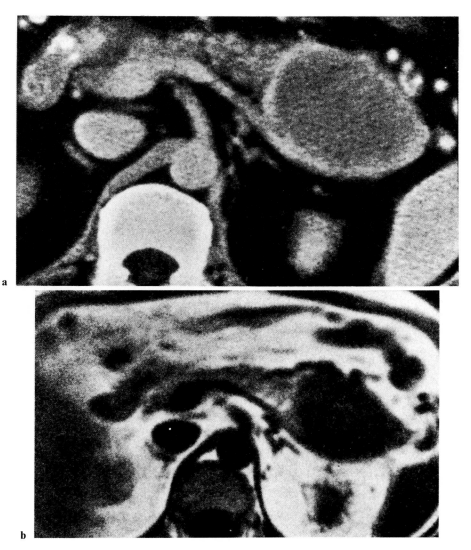

Fig. 31 a–d. Traumatic aneurysm of the splenic artery. The patient presented with persistent abdominal pain following abdominal trauma. **a** A low density mass in topography of the tail of the pancreas is observed. In the differential diagnosis, a pancreatic tumor was considered. **b** MRI showed the vascular nature of this mass. Note the flow void phenomenon in the mass, which appears in continuity with the splenic artery. **c** Duplex scanning with color Doppler showing the flow pattern during systole (*left*) and diastole (*right*). This finding is pathognomonic of a vascular abnormality of the splenic artery. **d** A splenic arteriogram showed an aneurysm of the splenic artery. Note the narrow neck of the aneurysm (*arrow*).

Following abdominal trauma, abdominal pain and/or melena warrants careful scrutiny of the pancreatic and peripancreatic region. Traumatic pancreatitis and false aneurysm should be sought. See Fig. 32 for additional recommendations

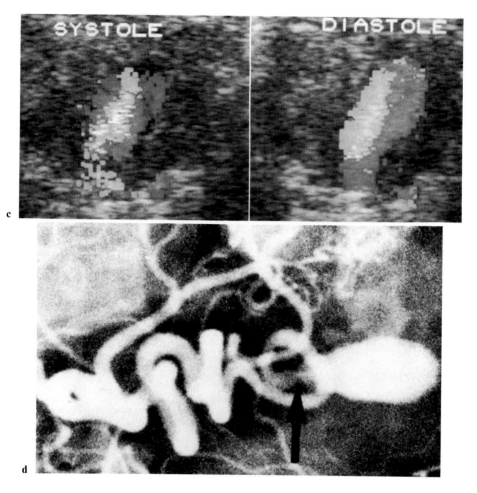

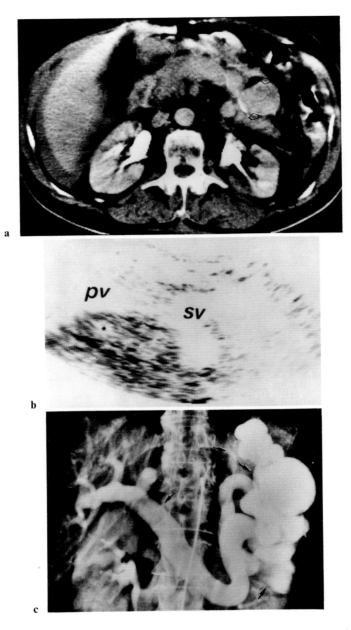

Fig. 32 a–c. Splenic arteriovenous fistula. Patient presented with left upper quadrant pain of uncertain etiology. **a** CT examination showed a mass in the topography of the tail of the pancreas (*arrowheads*). **b** US reveals enlarged splenic (*SV*) and portal (*PV*) veins. Note an anechoic mass distal to the splenic vein. **c** Venous late phase of selective splenic arteriogram. Note massively enlarged tributaries and enlarged splenic and portal veins. An arteriovenous fistula explains the pain in the left upper quadrant.

Noninvasive imaging modalities can be used to diagnose aneurysms and arteriovenous fistulae. US examination should be supplemented by Doppler technique

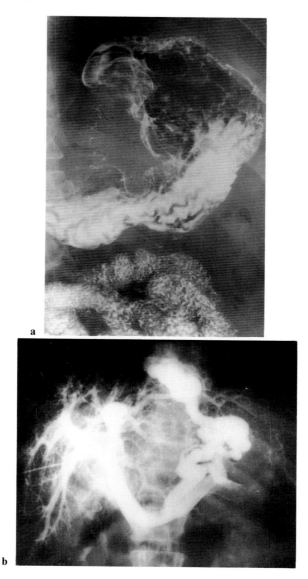

Fig. 33a, b. Gastric varices. **a** Mass effect in the fundus of the stomach and distorted folds. Carcinoma of the stomach was suspected. The patient had a history of chronic alcoholism and of gastrointestinal bleeding. **b** Transhepatic portography showed hepatofugal circulation, enlarged tributaries of the portal vein, gastric and esophageal varices. Apparent masses in the alimentary tract can be simulated by enlarged veins secondary to portal hypertension. A careful clinical history may suggest this possible etiology. Mucosal destructive patterns suggesting a neoplasia can be produced by inflammatory lesions, hemorrhage, and enlarged vessels

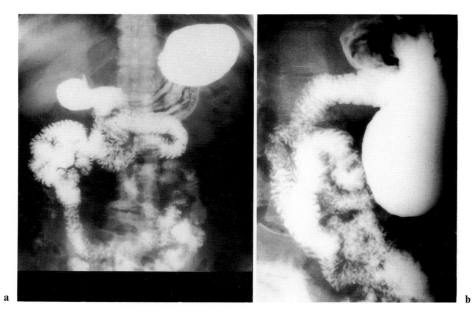

a   b

Fig. 34 a–f. Relocated bowel secondary to agenesis of the right kidney simulating a right paraduodenal hernia. This 50-year-old woman presented with nonspecific abdominal pain. **a, b** Frontal (**a**) and lateral (**b**) views of an upper GI series revealed an abnormal position of proximal jejunal loops. They projected dorsal to the second part of the duodenum and appeared in the right upper quadrant. **c** Frontal view of a barium enema. Note medial and high position of the ascending colon, which, with the proximal transverse colon, appears as a double barrel. **d** Representative film of a urogram. Note absence of the right kidney, enlarged normal left kidney, and numerous, proximal, jejunal loops in the right upper quadrant. **e** The earlier phase of the abdominal aortogram shows absence of the right kidney and of the right renal artery. **f** Late phase of the abdominal aortogram

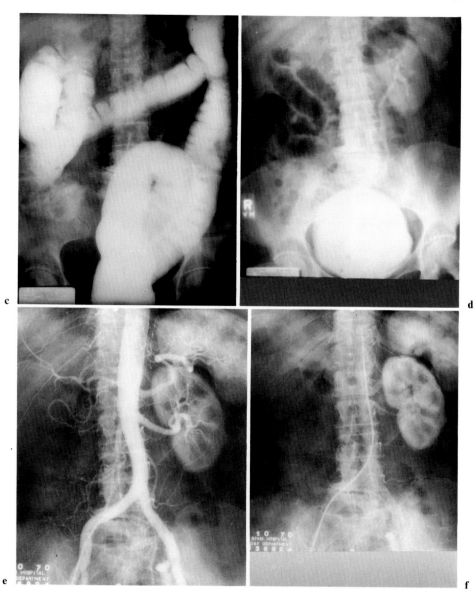

c

d

e

f

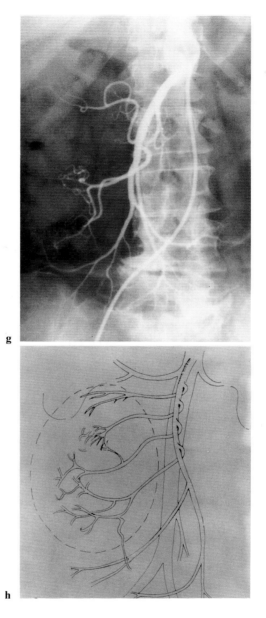

Fig. 34 g, h. Relocated bowel secondary to agenesis of the right kidney simulating a right paraduodenal hernia. **g** Selective superior mesenteric arteriogram. Due to the abnormal course of the proximal jejunal arteries, a right paraduodenal hernia was suspected. A lateral view of the superior mesenteric arteriogram was not obtained. **h** Diagram showing origin of proximal jejunal arteries in a patient with a right paraduodenal hernia. In this case the lateral view of the superior mesenteric arteriogram would have shown the *ventral* (not dorsal!) and right lateral direction of the proximal jejunal arteries. The right position of the jejunal loops was not related to an internal hernia but to agenesis of the right kidney. Organ relocation, in this case secondary to congenital absence of the kidney, can also occur following surgery or with ectopia

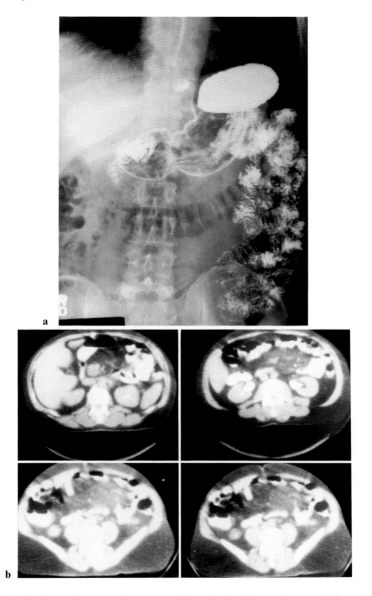

Fig. 35 a, b. Patient with retractile mesenteritis who had intermittent, colicky, abdominal pain and a palpable abdominal mass. **a** From an upper GI series. Note coalescence of proximal jejunal loops in the left upper quadrant and absence of small bowel loops in the central portion of the abdomen. **b** Representative images of a CT examination. The coalescence of small bowel loops is seen in the left upper quadrant and left flank region. A low density, central, mesenteric mass showing negative CT values suggestive of fat was observed. At surgery, tissue diagnosis revealed the presence of retractile mesenteritis. Table 4 (Appendix) describes the relationship of mesenteric panniculitis and retractile mesenteritis. The coalescence of small bowel loops simulated a left paraduodenal hernia. A clue to the diagnosis of retractile mesenteritis is the history of colicky adbominal pain and a CT examination revealing a fibrotic or fibroadipose mass associated with coalescence of small bowel loops

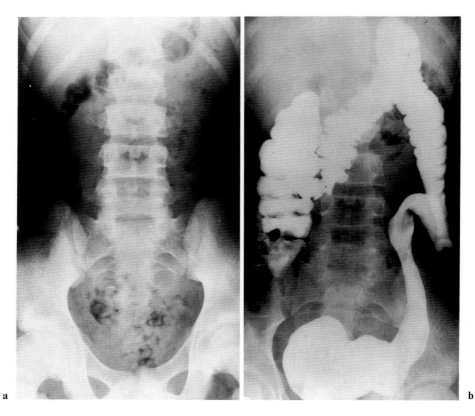

a   b

Fig. 36 a–d. Pelvic kidneys. This young man presented with a history of constipation and left lower quadrant pain. **a** Normal gas pattern. The outline of the kidneys is not visualized. **b** Barium enema revealed extrinsic compression of the sigmoid which has a spastic appearance and appears redundant. Note the medial position of the proximal descending colon and of the ascending colon. This should be a clue to the diagnosis of either renal agenesis or renal ectopia. **c** Oblique view following barium enema showing extrinsic compression of the proximal sigmoid and distal descending colon by the pelvic mass. **d** Representative film of an intravenous urogram. Two small pelvic kidneys appear in the pelvis. Note the bilateral short ureters.

The bowel occupying the usual position of the kidneys is indicative of either agenesis of the kidneys or renal ectopia. A urogram should be obtained. Tumors often arise from dysplastic and/or ectopic kidneys. Serial, noninvasive, imaging studies of the kidneys are recommended to detect the presence of a superimposed neoplasm on the anomalous kidney

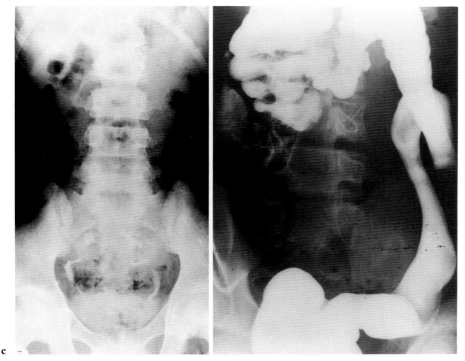

c   d

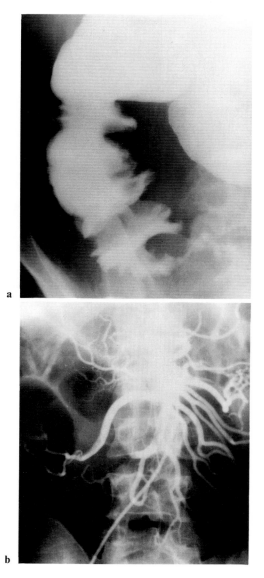

a

b

Fig. 37 a–d. Cecal infarction. This 64-year-old man had had a heart attack. Some 6 weeks after the heart attack, he developed acute right lower quadrant pain and had blood in the stools. **a** A barium enema was requested and revealed extensive mucosal distortion of the cecum and ascending colon. Thumbprinting is noted, particularly in the medial aspect of the cecum and ascending colon. **b** Earlier arterial phase and **c** late arterial phase of a superior mesenteric arteriogram. Note amputation of the right ileocolic artery and filling defects in the right colic branches. Note absence of vasa recta in topography of the cecum and ascending colon. The patient was treated conservatively and a repeat barium enema (**d**) shows a deformed cecum but restoration of the normal mucosal pattern. This is a classic example of ischemic colitis secondary to superior mesenteric artery embolism

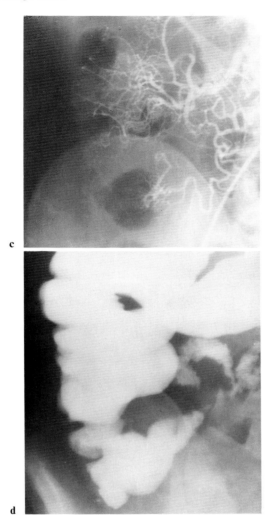

c

d

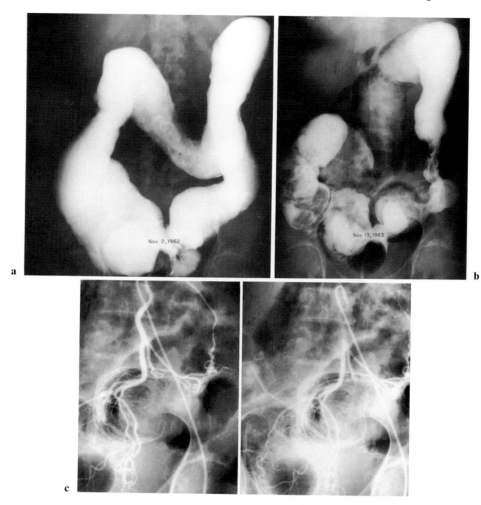

Fig. 38 a–c. Chronic ulcerative colitis with superimposed ischemic colitis. This 37-year-old woman gave a long history of chronic ulcerative colitis. **a** On November 2, 1962 she had a barium enema which showed signs of diffuse ulcerative colitis. A year later, she developed acute abdominal pain and **b** had another barium enema without preparation. Note a segmental lesion in the descending colon which simulates a carcinoma. At Grand Rounds, the Division of Gastroenterology and the Department of Surgery concluded that this was probably a complicating carcinoma superimposed on ulcerative colitis. We had been informed by the patient that, 1 month prior to admission, she had a barium enema that did not reveal any changes since the study of 1962. Therefore, we suspected the possibility of an acute lesion and requested postponement of surgery and authorization to do an angiographic examination. **c** Selective inferior mesenteric arteriogram. Note uniform hypervascularity in topography of the sigmoid and the distal descending colon. No vessels were seen in topography of the region where the segmental mucosal changes were observed in the barium enema

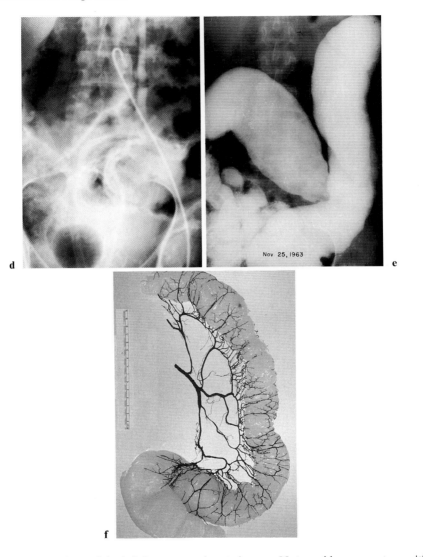

d–f. d Venous phase of the inferior mesenteric arteriogram. Note rapid venous return with filling of the inferior mesenteric vein (typical findings seen in ulcerative colitis). However, no veins appeared from the region where the segmental colonic lesion was observed. This suggested that the patient had ischemic colitis superimposed on ulcerative colitis. We asked that the barium enema be repeated. **e** Some 12 days following the initial study that revealed the segmental lesion, a barium enema showed disappearance of the constricting lesion and once again evidence of chronic ulcerative colitis. **f** Cast-corrosion of the veins of the sigmoid and descending colon. Note the small caliber of the veins that drain the large bowel.

Thromboses of small veins appear to be the cause of ischemic colitis in patients with inflammatory or neoplastic bowel disease. Often, proximal to a carcinoma, an area of ischemic colitis develops. It may simulate a very extensive tumor, when actually the tumor is small but the secondary ischemic colitis accounts for a larger lesion. Given a history of acute symptoms and an acute lesion, there should be conservative management, particularly when arteriography shows an ischemic process. Reversible bowel ischemic changes can be observed within a week or 10 days following ischemic insult

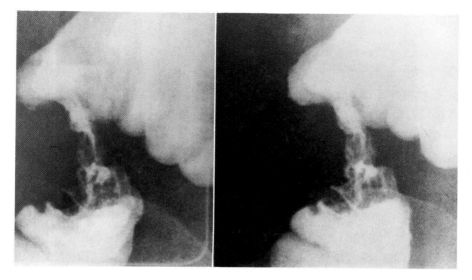

Fig. 39. Segmental ischemic colitis. Constricting lesion of the ascending colon simulating a carcinoma. The patient had a history of superior mesenteric artery embolism. Endoscopy and conservative management are recommended. Surgery may still be done if strictures develop

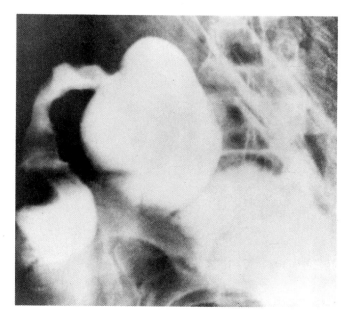

Fig. 40. Segmental ischemic colitis. Another proven case of segmental colitis simulating a carcinoma. Also, the patient had a history of superior mesenteric artery thrombosis

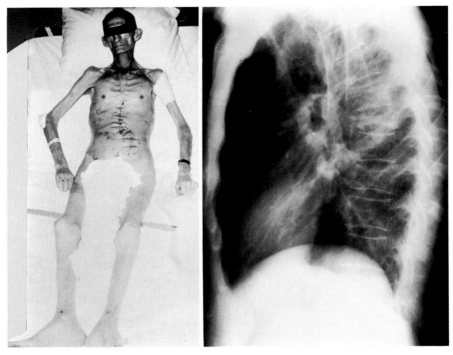

a   b

Fig. 41 a–e. Chronic intestinal ischemia simulating malignancy. **a** 48-year-old man who presented with profound cachexia, postprandial epigastric pain, vomiting, and diarrhea. This is a photograph of the patient 1 day after surgery. **b** Lateral chest radiograph showing diffuse osteopenia and a collapsed thoracic vertebra. **c** From an upper gastrointestinal series showing megaduodenum (see Appendix: Table 5), slow transit time, and disorder motor function of the small bowel. These findings suggested superior mesenteric artery syndrome, compressing the third part of the duodenum, and probably sprue. **d** From a small bowel series revealing stasis in the second part of the enlarged duodenum and disordered motor function of the small bowel. Crosby capsule biopsy of the small bowel showed findings suggesting sprue. At this time an abdominal malignancy was suspected. An arteriogram was requested. **e** Superior mesenteric artery injection showing slow flow and poor opacification of distal branches of the superior mesenteric artery and retrograde filling of the celiac trunk and antegrade opacification of the hepatic arteries (celiac artery steal syndrome)

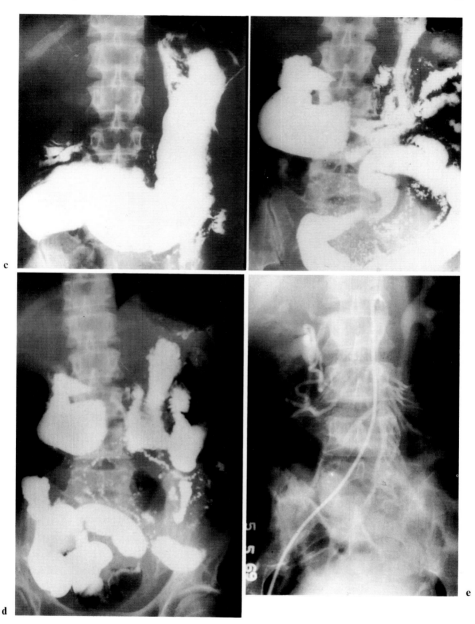

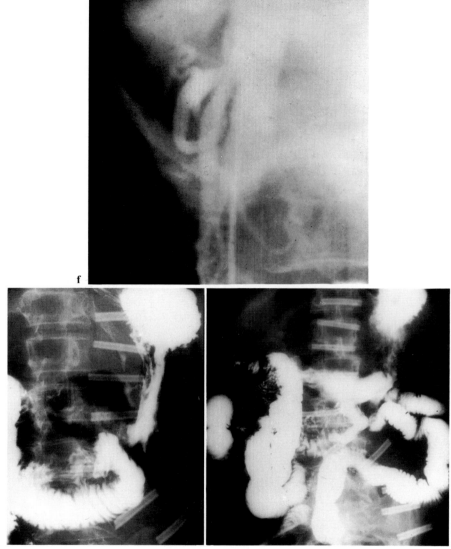

Fig. 41 f, g. Chronic intestinal ischemia simulating malignancy. **f** Lateral aortogram which reveals narrowing of the cephalic aspect of the celiac trunk suggestive of impression from the left crus of the diaphragm. This often occurs in asymptomatic individuals. At this time, although no evidence of malignancy was observed, a decision was made to perform an exploratory laparotomy, expecting to find a pancreatic neoplasm, a lymphoma, or some other type of malignancy. At surgery, no malignancy was found. The surgeon limited his procedure to exploration, to placing a patch on the celiac artery (a gradient of 40 mm was encountered between the aorta and the hepatic artery) and performing a duodenojejunostomy. Amazingly, the patient's pain disappeared after surgery. He started eating without vomiting. His diarrhea stopped and he progressively regained his weight. **g** A postoperative GI examination shows a return to a normal small bowel appearance, the disappearance of the megaduodenum, and no evidence of a slow transit time

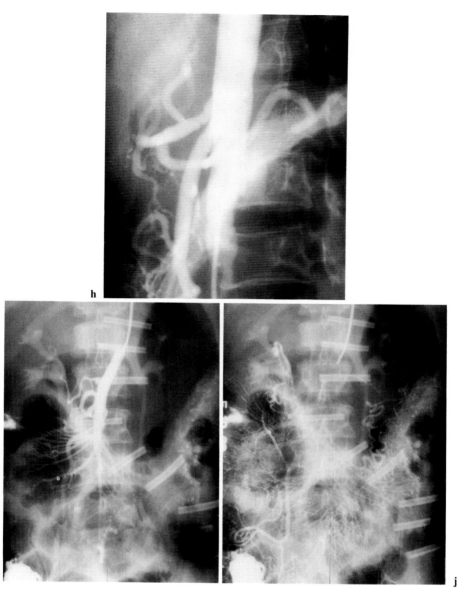

h–j. h A repeat aortogram shows a patent celiac trunk. **i, j** Superior mesenteric artery injection shows a normal rapid transit time with good opacification of the terminal branches of the superior mesenteric artery and a good blush of the small bowel (these were not present preoperatively). At this thime there was no evidence of celiac artery steal syndrome. Retrospectively, this pseudomalignancy was caused by celiac artery stenosis syndrome and Wilkie syndrome. The patient's abdominal pain appears to have been vasculogenic. He vomited because of his obstructed duodenum from the superior mesenteric artery syndrome. Celiac artery steal probably caused the chronic intestinal ischemia. Vomiting and poor intake of food caused a severe metabolic disorder, malnutrition, and cachexia

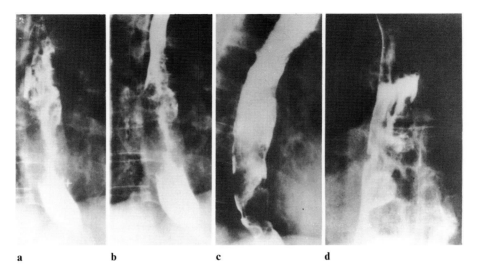

a   b   c   d

Fig. 42 a–d. Four examples of esophageal lesions mimicking a carcinoma. All were due to intramural hematomas of the esophagus

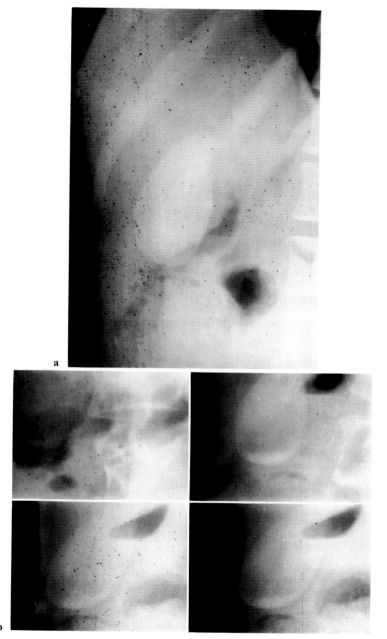

Fig. 43a, b. Pseudocalculi due to layering of contrast media. **a** An oral cholecystogram taken in the private office of a gastroenterologist. Note numerous artifacts. **b** Spot films of the study showing layering of the contrast material in the dependent portion of the gallbladder. This study was interpreted as possible gallstones. The patient underwent surgery on the basis of this examination and a normal gallbladder was found

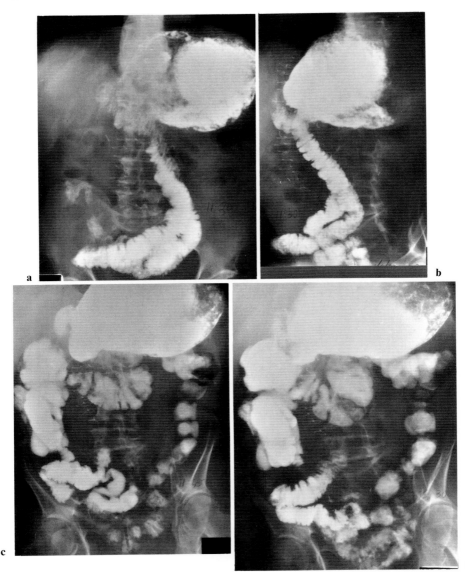

Fig. 44a–d. Iatrogenic short-bowel syndrome. The patient had a partial gastrectomy for peptic ulcer disease and, following surgery, developed chronic diarrhea. In the course of time, the patient's condition deteriorated and he eventually died of malnutrition. On postmortem examination, the stomach was found to have been anastomosed to the diatal ileum. This error should have been detected on post-operative GI examination. **a** Film of the abdomen taken immediately after the upper GI examination. Note distended gastric remnant and a long loop of bowel connecting the stomach to the distal small bowel. **b** A film taken 15 min later. Note opacification of distal small bowel loops and absence of opacification of the jejunum. **c** A film taken 15 min after the upper GI series. Note complete opacification of the colon. Barium appears retained in the stomach and in the distal small bowel. **d** Film taken 70 min after the upper GI examination. Note barium retained in the stomach, distal small bowel, and throughout the colon

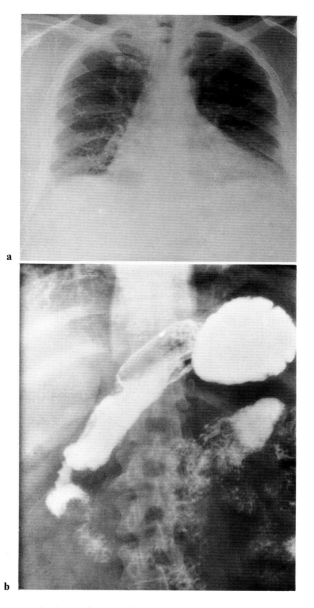

Fig. 45 a, b. Paravertebral pseudotumor in a very obese woman who presented with back pain. **a** A chest roentgenogram showed a discrete right paravertebral density. **b** From an upper GI series. Note the high position of the gastric antrum and a right paravertebral mass. This was initially interpreted as possibly being related to a pancreatic tumor, with extension to the right paravertebral region, or to a lymphoma. However, this patient had been gaining weight rather than losing weight

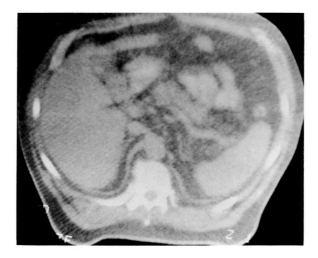

Fig. 45 c. Paravertebral pseudotumor in a very obese woman who presented with back pain. A CT revealed an abundance of fat in the retroperitoneum and no evidence of a pancreatic tumor. Spinal soft tissue densities are best assessed by CT. Fat can simulate tumor or a fluid collection in this region

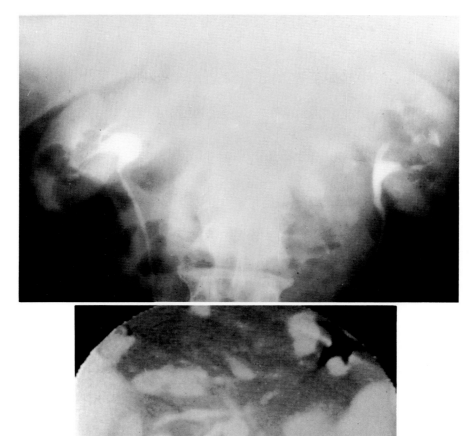

b

Fig. 46 a, b. Fat accumulation in the paravertebral region. Patient presented with nonspecific urinary tract abnormalities. **a** A urogram shows lateral displacement of the ureters. The diagnosis made at this time was that of a possible lymphoma, retroperitoneal sarcoma, or, less likely, an aneurysm of the aorta. **b** A CT of this region failed to demonstrate evidence of a tumor. The aorta was not enlarged. Abundance of fat in the retroperitoneum was the cause of the lateral displacement of the ureters. This patient did not have psoas hypertrophy, which can also produce displacement of the ureters

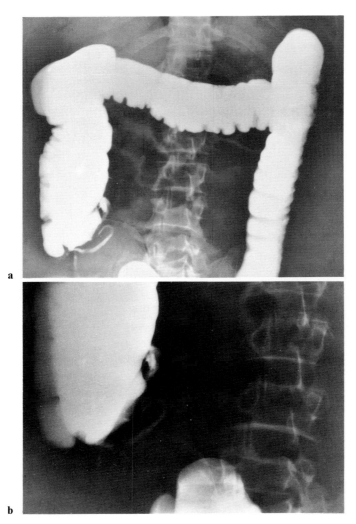

Fig. 47a–c. Psoas hypertrophy simulating extrinsic cecal mass. **a, b** Patient with nonspecific abdominal pain. **a** Barium enema shows a normal-appearing colon, except some flattening of the medial aspect of the cecum. Note visualization of a normal-appearing appendix. **b** Right posterior oblique film shows flattening of the medial aspect of the cecum. This was interpreted as a possible mass pressing on the cecum. **c** CT in a second patient shows marked hypertrophy of the psoas muscles. This patient had hypertrophied psoas muscles and paraspinal muscles as well. Note the compression of the cecum by the right psoas muscle

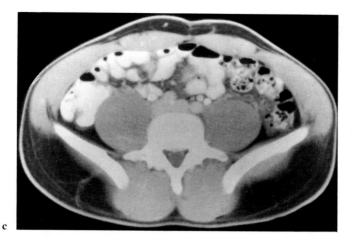

c

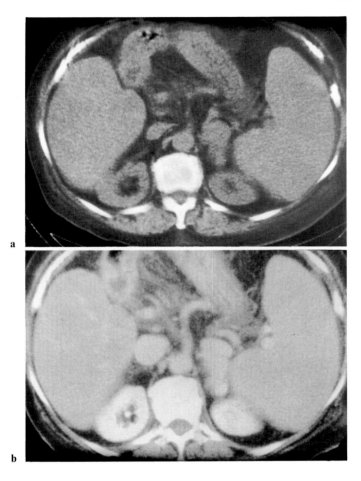

Fig. 48 a, b. The patient had chronic myelogenous leukemia and presented with splenomegaly and portal hypertension. **a** CT of the abdomen showed splenomegaly and a mass
in front of the left kidney simulating a large adrenal gland. **b** An enhanced CT study shows
opacification of juxtasplenic veins. Portal systemic collaterals were seen throughout the
abdomen. Varices simulated an enlarged adrenal gland

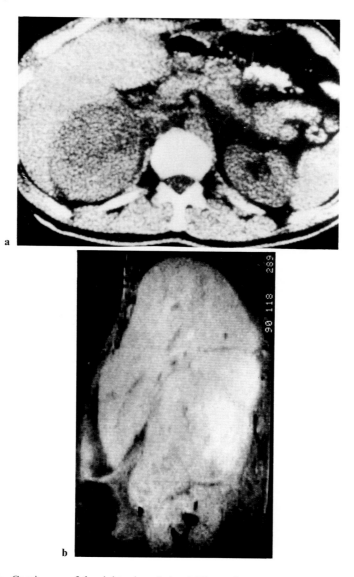

Fig. 49 a, b. Carcinoma of the right adrenal gland. The patient presented with a gynecomastia. **a** A CT of the abdomen showed a mass in the topography of the right lobe of the liver. **b** An MRI study (sagittal image) showed the liver (*L*) and the kidney (*K*) separated by a large polylobulated mass, which proved to be a carcinoma of the right adrenal gland. Cross-sectional imaging may reveal tumors of apparent liver origin. US examination and MRI often separate the mass from the liver. However, some pedunculated liver tumors, such as liver cell adenomas, can simulate juxtahepatic masses

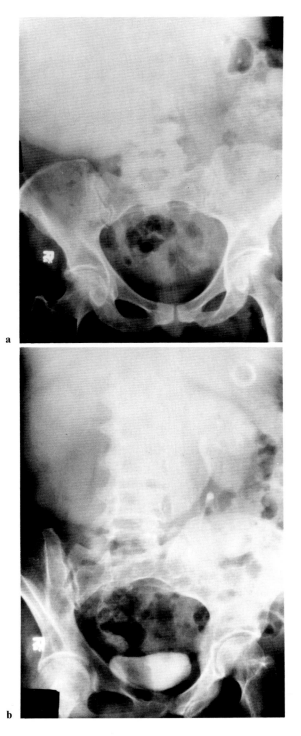

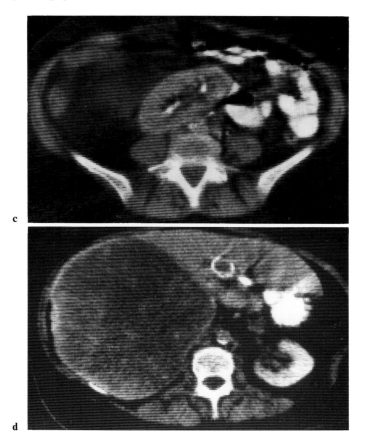

c

d

Fig. 50 a–d. Nonfunctioning pheochromocytoma of the right adrenal gland. **a** Mass in the right upper quadrant suspected of representing an enlarged liver. However, note the inferior convexity of the mass. Usually the outline of the liver produces a straight line or an inferior medial concavity. **b** Calcification in the left upper quadrant, the mass previously noted, and nonvisualization of the right kidney. However, on the left side, we noted a normal left kidney and a second pelvocalyceal system just below the left kidney. This is a left posterior oblique view of the intravenous urogram. **c** A CT examination showed the displaced right kidney in front of the spine. **d** A CT of the right upper quadrant revealed a low density large mass which proved to be a nonfunctioning pheochromocytoma. The calcific density was due to a gallstone! The liver had been displaced to the left and that is why the gallstone presented to the left of the midline.

Large retroperitoneal tumors grow towards the path of least resistance, which is ventrally. Cephalic growth may displace the liver. The tumors can be palpated anteriorly and to the right of the abdomen and simulate hepatomegaly. Noninvasive imaging modalities usually identify the anatomical location of the process. US in the sagittal plane can show the "sliding sign" of subhepatic tumors. The tumor can be separated, often from the lower margin of the liver, and appears displaced from the liver during inspiration and expiration. Tumors of the right kidney and of the right adrenal gland can be suspected by noting the sliding sign on sonography. Table 6 (Appendix) lists the most common liver calcifications

Appendix: Tables

The following tables 1–6 (cited in the text) provide additional information to the case studies illustrated and described in the atlas.

Table 1. Causes of veno-occlusive disease of the liver[a]

Hypercoagulable disorders (polycythemia vera)
Oral contraceptives
Plant alkaloids
Aflatoxin
Arsphenamine
Urethane
Ionizing radiation
Immunosuppressive and antineoplastic agents: azathioprine, 6-thioguanine
Bone marrow transplantation

[a] Nonthrombotic obliterative lesions of small centrilobular and sublobular hepatic veins.

Table 2. Causes of fatty liver

Obesity	Pregnancy
Alcoholism	Cushing's syndrome
Diabetes mellitus	High-dose steroid therapy
Pancreatic disease	Cystic fibrosis
Wilson's disease	Reye's syndrome
Kwashiorkor syndrome	Glycogen storage
Intestinal bypass	Acute hepatitis
Intravenous hyperalimentation	Idiopathic

Table 3. Systemic effects of renal cell carcinoma

Effect	Symptom	Patients (%)
General	Fever	17
	Malaise	
	Weight loss	
Hematologic	Anemia	33
	Elevated ESR	50
	Polycythemia	
Hepatic dysfunction		
Elevated serum phosphatase	Alkaline or acid	
Amyloidosis		3–5
Neurologic and neuropathic		
Endocrine	Hypertension (renin)	10–25
	Polycythemia (erythropoietin)	
	Hypercalcemia (parathormone)	
	Protein-losing enteropathy	
Immunologic	IgM paraprotein production	

Table 4. Relationship between mesenteric panniculitis and retractile mesenteritis [a]

Mesenteric panniculitis

Early phase:	Process limited to root of the mesentery of the small intestine
Morphology:	Mesentery of small intestine is markedly thickened; loss of fat lobulations; red-brown plaques represent fat necrosis
Histology:	Fat infiltrated by macrophages with an abundant foamy cytoplasm; widespread fat necrosis; ultimately fibrosis and calcification (fibrous lesions rare in early stages)
Comments:	Characterized largely by inflammation; synonyms are systemic Christian-Weber disease; isolated lipodystrophy; retractile mesenteritis

Retractile mesenteritis

Early phase:	Process is similar to mesenteric panniculitis but more extensive and more fibrotic; involves mesentery of the large intestine
Morphology:	Gradual appearance of an increasing number of intestinal adhesions
Comments:	Leads to adhesions and obstruction

[a] A case reported by Soergel, in which mesenteric panniculitis progressed to retractile mesenteritis, suggests the unity of these diseases. Clinical features of both diseases include: abdominal pain, nausea, vomiting, localized abdominal tenderness, and often a palpable abdominal mass.

Table 5. Causes of megaduodenum

1. Diabetes mellitus
2. Systemic lupus erythematosus
3. Scleroderma
4. Myxedema
5. Amyloidosis
6. Myotonic dystrophy
7. Chronic idiopathic intestinal obstruction
8. Superior mesenteric artery syndrome (Wilkie syndrome)
9. Cast's syndrome

Table 6. The most common liver calcifications

Inflammatory	
Infection	Pyogenic liver abscess; brucellosis; tuberculosis; syphilis; histoplasmosis; coccidoidmycosis
Infestation	Amebic abscess; hydatid disease; *Ascaris lumbricoides; Armillifer armillatus; Opisthorchis sinensis;* cysticercosis; filiariasis; guinea worm; *Paragonimus westermani;* toxoplasmosis
Neoplasms	
Benign	Cavernous hemangioma
Primary malignant	Hepatoblastoma; hepatocellular carcinoma; cholangiocarcinoma; hemangioendothelioma
Metastatic	Lymphoma
Nonparasitic cysts	
Post-traumatic hepatoma	
Intrahepatic calculi	
Gaucher's disease	
Shock liver	
Vascular	Portal; hepatic artery; IVC thrombus; malformation; atherosclerotic lesion
Capsular	Alcoholic cirrhosis; pyogenic infection; pseudomyxoma peritonei; meconium peritonitis; lipoid granulomatosis; barium granulomatosis
Increase radiodensity without calcification	Alcoholic cirrhosis; hemochromatosis; siderosis; thorotrast injection

M. Viamonte Jr.,
Mount Sinai Medical Center,
Miami Beach, FL

Errors in Chest Radiography

1991. VI, 135 pp. 102 figs. in 296 sep. illus.
4 tabs. Softcover DM 90,–
ISBN 3-540-52906-3

Why are mistakes made in chest radiography?
Many errors are caused simply by wrong technique or faulty interpretation. How can a specialist
avoid making such mistakes? By recognizing the
reasons for past mistakes.

Dr. Viamonte has collected many such cases, particularly of bronchial cancer, during thirty years of
experience.
He distinguishes between errors of omission,
which occur most often, errors of commission,
and errors caused by a lack of relevant clinical
history. The original
radiograph is presented
thus challenging the
reader to recognize the
abnormality correctly.
Every practicing radiol-
ogist can learn from
the cases and pitfalls
presented in this book.

Springer-Verlag
Berlin
Heidelberg
New York
London
Paris
Tokyo
Hong Kong
Barcelona
Budapest

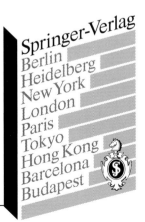

D. Beyer, Cologne,
U. Mödder, University of Düsseldorf

Diagnostic Imaging of the Acute Abdomen

A Clinico-Radiologic Approach

With contributions by numerous experts
With a Foreword by H. Pichlmaier
Translated from the German by T. C. Telger
1988. XV, 453 pp. 250 figs., containing 680 separate
illus. Hardcover DM 196,– ISBN 3-540-17520-2

The acute abdomen is one of the most frequent, most
dangerous and most difficult problems that the diagnostic radiologist has to deal with. This comprehensive
manual presents a clinico-radiologic approach to the
use of diagnostic imaging techniques for acute abdominal conditions. Imaging techniques, radiologic symptoms and clinical conditions are treated separately.
This lucid format, together with a detailed subject
index, offer the reader a quick and reliable reference
aid in daily practice. The text is clearly structured and
concise in style, and provides helpful practical hints,
including discussion of diagnostic
pitfalls. It is supported by a
wealth of illustrations cover-
ing native diagnosis, ultrasonography, computer
tomography and
angiography.

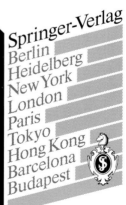

Springer-Verlag
Berlin
Heidelberg
New York
London
Paris
Tokyo
Hong Kong
Barcelona
Budapest

Distribution rights for Japan:
Nankado

Prices are subject to change
without notice.